# why i don't hide my *freckles* anymore

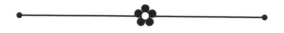

# why i don't hide my *freckles* anymore

*Perspectives on True Beauty*

*Edited by*
LaNae Valentine and
Lisa Tensmeyer Hansen

DESERET
BOOK

Salt Lake City, Utah

"The Beauty underneath the Surface," by S. Michael Wilcox is reprinted by permission from S. Michael Wilcox, *Walking on Water and Other Classic Messages* (Salt Lake City: Deseret Book, 2011), 146–47.

**Library of Congress Cataloging-in-Publication Data**

Why I don't hide my freckles anymore : perspectives on true beauty / edited by LaNae Valentine and Lisa Tensmeyer Hansen.

    pages cm

  Collection of short essays by female Brigham Young University students and others on the messages modern culture sends about physical beauty.

  Includes bibliographical references.

  ISBN 978-1-60907-806-5 (paperbound)

  1. Body image. 2. Self-esteem in women. 3. Feminine beauty (Aesthetics)—Psychological aspects. 4. Beauty, Personal—Psychological aspects. I. Valentine, LaNae, editor of compilation. II. Hansen, Lisa, 1958– editor of compilation. III. Brigham Young University. Women's Services and Resources, sponsoring body.

  BF697.5.B63W49 2013

  306.4'613—dc23                        2013034115

Printed in the United States of America
Edwards Brothers Malloy, Ann Arbor, MI

10  9  8  7  6  5  4  3  2  1

# Contents

## Contents

# Contents

# Contents

# Contents

# Introduction

What woman doesn't want to be beautiful—or at least pretty? Especially when she's been taught it's the most important thing about her. Is there a woman out there who actually feels good in her body and likes how she looks? A woman's relationship with her body is one of the most important relationships she'll ever have. If that relationship isn't working, everything else is harder.

The idea for this book developed from a need we saw among our Brigham Young University students who, like women everywhere, sometimes fall prey to dangerous ideas about beauty, bodies, and self-worth.

As much as we try to protect our children and ourselves from toxic messages and practices in our culture, we can't help but be affected by them. Girls today are growing up in a dangerous, sexualized, media-saturated culture where they face incredible pressure to be thin, sexy, and physically perfect. These messages tell us our natural bodies are deficient; our faces are not pretty without make-up; our hair should be colored, straightened, curled, and tamed; we shouldn't sweat; and our clothing must be restrictive and revealing. These messages limit our freedom to be our true selves and make us feel unsafe in our own bodies.

We at BYU Women's Services and Resources want to play a role in promoting a culture less complicated and more nurturing, less objectifying and more growth-producing. We want to enhance a woman's sense of her body as a haven of safety, care, and respectful stewardship. BYU students were invited to write about coming to a place of peace and acceptance regarding how they look. Later, we extended the invitation to faculty, staff and other women who frequent the Women's Services and Resources website and blog. We even recruited the valuable insights of a couple of brave men to contribute to our cause.

Reflection and writing allow us see ourselves and others more truthfully, more compassionately. Our personal experiences challenge the illusions of the culture. We begin to see how unfulfilling and shallow the messages are. We sense a newfound strength and power to stand up to false standards of self-worth and refuse to allow ourselves to be merchandise in the marketing of beauty. Real beauty isn't merely decorative; its primary function is to connect—to connect our innermost beings to one another and to the world around us. Real beauty does not divide or diminish us—it opens and inspires us. It is not only possible but natural to live peacefully in our body, to be comfortable in our own skin, for each of us to love our bodies and find ourselves beautiful.

As you read these essays, we hope you will feel nourished and blessed by the wisdom and truth in them. We hope these stories will help you in your own journey to capture the reality of true beauty.

LaNae Valentine, editor

---

NOTE

The compilers wish to thank Brooke Beecher Schultz for her vision and help in gathering many of the pieces included in this collection, and also thank all who contributed stories and essays that have enriched our experience of beauty.

❀

# Cosmetic Surgery for the Heart

## LaNae Valentine

*It is only with one's heart that one can see clearly.*
*What is essential is invisible to the eye.*

—Antoine de Saint-Exupéry[1]

In the second grade, when I got my first pair of eyeglasses my mother said, "My little girl isn't pretty anymore." A few years later, my brother told me I had ugly teeth and called me a rude name.

Years later, I overheard a boy I was dating say to his friend that he thought I was cute except he thought my nose was too big. Another boy who was teaching me to dive commented that I looked great in a swimsuit, barring my large hips. Yet another boy told me I was a fun person but that I didn't have much on top. I took all of these comments about my body and tucked them away in my heart. They have stuck with me over the years and negatively affected the way I see and feel about myself.

---

**LaNae Valentine** *is the director of Women's Services and Resources at Brigham Young University. When she's not working to support, connect, and empower women she enjoys visiting family and friends, cycling through Utah's back roads and canyons, cooking, reading, and doing yoga.*

Eventually I got contact lenses and had my teeth fixed, which helped me feel better about myself. Yet, whenever I looked in the mirror I still saw a big nose, large hips, and a flat chest. I habitually wore long sweaters and shirts to cover my hips, padded bras to enhance my chest, and avoided wearing swimsuits like the plague.

These experiences have taught me that words can have a deep impact on people—for good or bad. Why do those careless, negative words seem to stick like super-strength adhesive while the positive ones slide off like soft butter? Why do we so willingly believe the negative words? Researchers say we need to have a ratio of at least ten or more positive interactions to counter every negative one. Left unattended, the negatives can cloud and color every aspect of our life.

It's tempting to believe that these negative beliefs about my body would be resolved if I could have nose surgery to make my nose smaller, liposuction to reduce my hips, and implants to augment my breasts. Then I would finally feel good about myself, right? Those modifications might have a temporary effect, but none of these surgeries would be enough. The surgery required must go deeper—it must cut to the heart where my shame resides.

Often our bodies become the scapegoat for all of the things we don't like about ourselves. Somehow it's easier to blame our bodies for our bad feelings than to look deeper. If we have an inner conviction of our worth, negative words might sting temporarily, but they won't stick. We won't believe them, we won't be so concerned about what people think of us, and we won't feel compelled to perfect our bodies to prove our worth.

The shame at the core of a negative body image is not an easy thing to shed. Shame is a full mind-body-heart emotion, an intensely painful feeling and belief that we are so flawed we are not worthy of love and acceptance. One writer described it as the silent hemorrhaging of the soul.[2] Shame makes us go into hiding. It prevents us from getting close to others for fear of disapproval or rejection. We become perfectionists, compelled to prove our worth. The surgery needed to heal these wounds must remove the cancer of self-loathing that permeates every aspect of my being. A radical change in how I see and feel about myself is required—a surgery not to transform my nose or breasts, but my heart.

Where can I go for such a surgery? I don't think it's a one-time event under the surgeon's scalpel, although I wish it were. The change of heart comes gradually as I open myself to trust and love—knowing the very thing that closed my heart in the first place might happen again. But better a broken heart than an impenetrable one. Better a heart that is bruised and tender than a heart safely locked in a dark, motionless coffin.

The change of heart comes gradually as I unwrap my layers of protection, refusing to engage in busy, numbing habits and allowing myself to connect to others—all of which bring with them the possibility of pain. But pain is good, a sign that my heart is coming to life. No more hiding, no more performing. This letting go of control brings up fears of loss, rejection, and abandonment. As I expose all the hidden places of my soul, I learn that my vulnerabilities make me real, that I am not alone, that being real is what connects us and love, not competition, is the better way.

This intimacy with myself and others takes time—time for rest, time for walks, time for quiet reflection, time to tune into my inner knowing. As I become intimate with myself, I discover my connection with others and the Divine. I learn there is strength in stillness. I learn to trust the voice which beckons *this is the way*. I recognize that I am loved and always have been.

Softly and gently I come to the awareness that who I am is enough. What a relief I feel when I sit with the possibility that I am enough. Can it really be true that I am not what I do or what

I produce or what I accomplish? I will sit with this feeling of being enough and let it heal my heart. I will embrace God's many creations of beauty—of which I am one.

---

## NOTES

1. Antoine de Saint-Exupéry, *The Little Prince* (Ware, UK: Wordsworth Editions Ltd., 1995), 82.
2. See Sarah Ban Breathnach, *Something More: Excavating Your Authentic Self* (New York: Hachette, 1998).

# I Walk in Beauty

## Cynthia L. Hallen

My life's pilgrimage has been a quest for Beauty. Not the beauty of the world, but *Beauty*. No English word captures the essence of my quest, but my Navajo teacher taught me a word that does: *Hózhó*. In the Navajo language, *shaa hózhó* means, "I am in tune with the Spirit; I am in harmony with Creation; I walk in Beauty."

In traditional Navajo culture, girls make the transition to womanhood by participating in a ceremony called the Beauty Way. Each morning before dawn, the young maiden runs toward the east to greet the sun. When the dawn arrives, she walks back home, singing:

> I walk in beauty, yes I do, yes I do.
> I talk in beauty, yes I do, yes I do.
> I dream of beauty, just for you and only you.
> Hey yah, hey yah, hey yo.

**Cynthia L. Hallen** *is a philologist by profession and a poet by nature. Her family abides in and around Phoenix, Arizona, while she resides in the green pastures and still waters of Springville, Utah. She defends the sanctity of life and traditional marriage. Her bliss is ice skating to the tunes of Owl City.*

I write in beauty, yes I do, yes I do.
I read in beauty, yes I do, yes I do.
I weave of beauty, just for you and only you.
Hey yah, hey yah, hey yo.

Each young woman knows herself as Beauty, carries herself in Beauty, takes her cue from Nature, and gives back to the world in Beauty. Indeed, Beauty is her stewardship. Like the song of a bird, Beauty is "thrilling toil."

> The Bird her punctual music brings
> And lays it in its place—
> Its place is in the Human Heart
> And in the Heavenly Grace—
> What respite from her thrilling toil
> Did Beauty ever take—
> But Work might be electric Rest
> To those that Magic Make
>
> —Emily Dickinson[1]

God has given all women Beauty, which has been placed like birdsong in our "Human Heart" by "Heavenly Grace." I am accountable for the songs placed there, be they one, two, or five songs. I deceive myself if I deny the portion of Beauty the Lord has placed in my heart or bury it underneath jealousy, self-pity, or vanity.

When I consider my personal songs of Beauty, I take note. I have inherited bad cholesterol but good bones, crooked teeth but a bright smile, a small chest but long legs, a receding chin but a keen mind, nervous anxiety but boundless energy. Who am I to begrudge the unique combination of elements passed down to me from the love of my ancestors? Some of them were, perhaps, unattractive people who worked lifetimes in farm and field, suffering in wars and troubles, growing old early, but they had Beauty too.

> They wore rags, ate acorns, went barefoot, lived in huts and hovels. . . . [Yet their] weather-beaten faces, their wens and goiters and crooked backs are to be seen in old Flemish paintings.[2]

Today, these cherished ancestors reside in the Spirit World, anticipating the Second Coming of the Savior. And "on that glad day all distinctions between high and low, rich and poor" will cease.[3] Despite any limitations experienced in life, they will run forward to meet the Son, and soon they will walk home with Him, singing celestial songs of redeeming love, perfected and glorified in body and spirit.

Some years ago, I stopped coloring my hair. Three things convinced me: (1) The effect of harsh chemicals on my sensitive skin; (2) associating with temple ordinance workers beautifully adorned by gray hair; and (3) a chance meeting with a man I had admired for years. He had been my family home evening brother twenty years earlier. I noticed the snow of middle age resting gently on his dark brown hair. If "the beauty of old men is the gray head" (Proverbs 20:29), then I too could seek Beauty in the authenticity of my age.

The Greek word for beauty is *hōra*, meaning "in due time." What is more beautiful than a gift or reward that arrives just when it should? Our words spoken at just the right time are Beauty; our actions that help heal another's pain are Beauty, given at just the right time.

What does it matter if I am despised or rejected because another person thinks I am not beautiful enough? The Lord "hid not [his] face from shame and spitting" (see Isaiah 50:6). Why should I hide mine? When I see the Lord, I shall be drawn to Him because of His loving kindness toward me, not because of His resplendent physical appearance.

My body is Beautiful simply because it is a temple in the plan of salvation. If I seek the Lord, He "will beautify the meek with salvation" (Psalm 149:4). He makes my feet "beautiful upon the mountains" (Isaiah 52:7). He has appointed unto me "beauty for ashes" and "the oil of joy for mourning" (Isaiah 61:3). He covers my mortal soul with immortality, crowning me with jewels of virtue (see Isaiah 61:10).

Someday I will see as I am seen . . . in Beauty. I will do more than walk in Beauty. I will *be* Beauty. *Hey yah, hey yah, hey yo.*

---

## NOTES

1. Emily Dickinson, "The bird her punctual music brings" (J 1585 / F 1556), *The Poems of Emily Dickinson: Variorum Edition*, ed. Ralph W. Franklin (Cambridge, MA: The Belknap Press of Harvard University Press, 1998). Reprinted by permission of the publishers and the Trustees of Amherst College from THE POEMS OF EMILY DICKINSON: VARIORUM EDITION, edited by Ralph W. Franklin, Cambridge, Mass.: The Belknap Press of Harvard University Press, Copyright © 1998 by the President and Fellows of Harvard College. Copyright © 1951, 1955, 1979, 1983 by the President and Fellows of Harvard College.
2. Robert M. Adams, *The Land and Literature of England: A Historical Account* (New York: Norton, 1982), 68, 69.
3. Ibid, 69.

❀

# I Collect Bodies in My Basement

## Jana Winters Parkin

I collect bodies in my basement.

And I feel good about it.

Every summer I take the kids to the pool. They adore what I avoid: Exposure. To the water, the sunshine. To other people.

While they frolic and splash, I seek cover in the shade, fully clothed, attempting to lose myself in a novel. I note the irony of isolating myself at a pool labeled *community*. When I face the thought of exposing my physical flaws, my body feels more like a prison than a temple.

Nearly lulled to sleep by the afternoon heat, I squint toward the pool. Hiding behind my sunglasses, I see people enjoying the water. Wonderful people, in every shape, size, and color—some rotund and Rubenesque, others elongated like a Modigliani. Observing with my artist's eye, I appreciate the distinctive beauty of each one.

---

**Jana Winters Parkin** *spent most of her adult life in Los Angeles, where she and her husband ran a successful design firm while raising three spirited children. When they moved to Utah, Jana abandoned her "designer to the rich and famous" career for a more peaceful regimen: painting, hiking, and writing. She has recently overcome her pathological fear of swimsuits.*

Leaning into the sunshine, I dig through the beach bag for the sketchbook I brought from my basement studio. Quickly, rhythmically, sometimes without even looking at the paper, I begin to draw. In fleeting strokes I try to capture all of those life-filled bodies: Families strolling by. Mothers standing, hips cocked to one side, talking to complete strangers. Grandmothers stooping over large, unwieldy beach bags. Children sliding and laughing. Little ones wrapped in bright-colored towels shivering in the sun. I suspend time, movement, and space as I collect these gestures one at a time in my sketchbook. *I want to save them.*

The imperfect bodies are the most interesting to an artist. The rolls and folds create elegant forms. I notice that a pregnant woman's belly mirrors her toddler's, and I contemplate the connection. I study the variety of proportions and find that none is wrong.

Having cast myself to this far-off corner in relative darkness, I suddenly feel ashamed. Not so much of my body, but of the way I hide it, enshroud it, and even loathe it. I recognize that, in my reluctance to join the others in the pool, I've fallen prey to the ultimate body snatcher. He and his legions covet my flawed, mortal frame—and cheat me into devaluing my greatest treasure.

I am in awe of the souls who courageously parade their corpulence without inhibition. They don't mind being exposed and vulnerable in swimsuits; they're simply enjoying the water and the sunshine and the community. *As they should.*

I yearn to develop an artist's eye—*the Creator's view*—toward my own imperfect body. I'm slowly learning to rejoice in my own ripples and curves rather than lamenting the loss of the hard body of my twenties. It's easier to love the pillow of padding on my belly when I remember how I earned it: creating life, giving birth. I think about how cold and dark my studio downstairs is and wonder: Were I to pull out of my basement the beautiful bodies

I've collected in my sketchbooks—my creations celebrating *His* creations—might I somehow pull myself into that light as well? Perhaps then I could escape this notion of a prison and celebrate my body for the temple it is . . . both for how it's shaped, and for the divinity it houses.

# Was It Something I Said?

## Jennifer Blaylock

When I was a girl my mother told me this:

"I'm glad my daughters aren't beautiful."

(She had four of them.)

"My daughters are interesting and smart and clever instead."

We were sitting at a stoplight at Stapley and University.

I don't remember where we were going.

I had heard this in little bits and pieces all my life, but somehow—maybe my age, maybe the stillness of the car, maybe the car itself as holding cell for an unwitting prisoner—this time especially, the words stung. And penetrated deep into my soul.

My mother was always pointing out who was beautiful; not just pretty, but *really* beautiful: My tall, blonde, confident aunt with high cheekbones and deep brown eyes—oh, yes, movie star beautiful; someone in my peer group at church, who was not especially nice to me—yes, she was beautiful too; a smattering of

**Jennifer Blaylock** *is an avid recreational beachcomber and road trip aficionado. She is a proud member of the I'm-writing-a-book-in-my-hard-to-find-spare-time club and also moonlights as a writer for an Internet marketing company. She lives with her husband and five children on the East Coast.*

beautiful cousins; the whole population of Czech girls, after returning from a humanitarian trip. The list went on.

Here's what I knew about myself: I had a thin, long face and I didn't look good without bangs.

My mother told me so.

(Incidentally, it was seven years and three children into my marriage before I finally threw the "must wear bangs" rule out the window. I actually tried my absolute best to *never* let my husband see me with my bangs pulled off my forehead. I laugh now. What wasted energy.)

My mother is not a wretched woman.

I think in her own way she meant for that first statement to be a compliment: "Honey, I am so proud of the brilliant, independent, interesting person you're becoming. You are so much more than your beautiful face."

But somehow, by default of my tender age, I missed that.

And maybe no one ever told her she was beautiful.

How could I be so hideous (my words now) and unattractive to the one person in the world who was supposed to love me best?

The explanation: It must be true.

Sometimes, now as an adult, my mother will tell me I look nice.

It's sad—I think she really might think so, but it's hard for me to believe it.

My poor husband, he tells me I am beautiful, and he tells me all he sees when he looks into my face. He tells me officially now he's "had me" longer than my parents, so all those insecurities should be undone.

But scars are scars, and they run deep.

So, in my mothering, maybe I've gone overboard in the opposite direction.

I think my children are beautiful, and I tell them every chance I get.

Truly, they are more than likely to hear it at least once a day.

Am I raising delusional, stuck-up children, full of pride and conceit?

(If you knew my children, I think you would say not.)

They have their insecurities and doubts just like everyone else.

Am I raising children who are focused more on looks rather than character, integrity, and intelligence?

(If you knew my children, I think you would say not.)

Am I raising children who are disproportionately preoccupied with the way that others see them, rather than how they see themselves?

(If you knew my children, I think you would say not.)

Maybe the key is not comparing their faces to anyone else's.

It's not about my favorite color of eyes, or a nose that is just so, or my preference to a particular shape of face, or the wave or texture of their hair. It's not about telling them I think they are more beautiful than their friends.

It's the smile that melts my heart that is beautiful; the one with the chapped lips and crooked teeth or the deep dimple right in the middle of a cheek. I tell them *that* is beautiful to me.

It's the twinkle in their eyes as they tell me a funny anecdote; the depth in their eyes as they share a concern; the kindness in their eyes as they help someone and don't even know I'm watching; the way the light hits their eyes and makes them sparkle like a thousand stars when they tell me about something good that happened to them that day. I tell them *that* is beautiful to me.

It's the way their brow furrows in concentration, or the faraway look of a great ponder, or an amused smile at that really funny part in the book—so absorbed in the reading that they are oblivious to having an audience. I tell them *that* is beautiful to me.

It's the way their eyelashes lay in a shadowy smudge across their cheeks when they close their eyes to pray or when they've fallen asleep. How that one lock of hair keeps finding its way to a troublesome spot and requires an absentminded, automatic brush of the hand . . .

They watch me drink in every last inch of their faces, and they know that I love what I see—because I tell them so.

Sometimes I worry. Have I told them they are beautiful *too much*?

Due to circumstances not of our choosing, four years ago we plucked them up from comfort and familiarity and set them down in a place that was more than a little prickly and cold and culturally different from anything they had ever been exposed to. Welcome to a taste of the refiner's fire, my babies.

It has been full of challenges, culture shock, and loneliness.

But children are incredible.

They survive.

I am so amazed at their strength and courage and resilience.

And if the knowledge that their mama thinks they are beautiful has helped them to weather these early thunderstorms of life, if the knowledge that their mama thinks they're beautiful has given them the quiet confidence to get back up when they are pushed down, if the knowledge that their mama thinks they're beautiful helps them on their journey to discovering who they are and all they can accomplish, then I'm happy to have given it.

And I'm glad it was something I said.

# Beauty Is a Virtue

## Eve Sonali Scorup

Hello. My name is Eve Scorup, and I am in the sixth grade. I see Beauty as a virtue like Honesty or Integrity. But unlike other virtues, beauty is given to *everyone* by God, and so it exists in each of us.

There is beauty in me, too. What is it? I'll start with my personality. I am kind, loving, patient, tenderhearted, honest, content, and grateful. In academics, I am willing to learn. I am very good at thinking things through and figuring things out, like analogies and theories. I am good at memorizing songs, poems, stories, and scripts for plays and skits. I write stories, poems, songs, essays, and reports. I enjoy journaling and public speaking. I am good at making friends, and I am a very good friend. I have fun, and I love being with people. I am helpful at home by taking care of my siblings and cooking (which I am very good at!).

Who are some people who have helped me discover my inner beauty? My parents gave me the middle name Sonali, which

---

**Eve Sonali Scorup's** *favorite hobbies are reading, playing music (especially piano), and writing pieces she hopes will be bestsellers when she fulfills her dream of being an author. She also enjoys hanging out with friends, learning new things, and being with her family.*

means "beautiful and kind" in Hindi. My mom gave me the nickname "Sweet Pea," referring to my sweet and gentle nature. My dad recently said I didn't need makeup to look pretty. My extended family calls me kind and beautiful. At church, Sister Ferguson said I looked nice and had a shiny glow around my face. My friends say I am nice and fun. These people help me to recognize my inner beauty by reminding me that they love me for me.

Beauty is a virtue that we discover in ourselves as we live in harmony with who we are. It is a virtue that we express as we live genuinely with other people.

# Capturing the Rainbow

## Karin Brown

There was still a trace of rain in the air as I drove south on the interstate. The road stretched like a ribbon straight to the horizon. Fortresslike mountains reached high on the east while a flat, gray lake bordered the west. Heavy gray rainclouds hovered above. A perfect painting hung in the frame of my windshield. The beautiful display of color arched through the sky, appearing to rest on the road ahead of me.

*Rainbows are beautiful, no matter the day*, I thought. Sometimes the backdrop is a gray sky. Sometimes the air sparkles like diamonds with leftover water droplets from a sudden summer shower. Sometimes the rainbow arches the entire sky, and other times you catch just a glimpse of the colorful crescent—a smattering of color between straggling clouds. Many people have attempted to capture the elusive beauty of rainbows in art, photography, or words. But no one captures the rainbow itself.

---

**Karin Brown**, *from Woods Cross, Utah, started out as a self-proclaimed gypsy world traveler until she met her husband, who inspired her to finish her English degree at Brigham Young University, plant roots in Utah, and raise a family, which now includes five children. She enjoys reading, hiking, music, and dancing in her kitchen when no one is looking.*

As I drove down the highway that day, keeping an eye on the rainbow ahead, my heart was filled with longing for my daughter to know that she is as stunning as a rainbow. "Oh, Sydney," I might say, "a rainbow isn't beautiful because of its shape and color, it's beautiful because it was created by God. Its meaning is even greater than its beauty. It holds promise of future love and deliverance. It reflects not only light but divine goodness. Just like you.

"Sydney, the world tells you that beauty springs from shape and color, that the reflection that matters is the reputation of your accomplishments. However, that kind of beauty is as unattainable as grasping a rainbow. The more you seek it, the harder it is to hold. Your true beauty is that you were created by God.

"Sydney, when you see your body, your mind, and your heart, see the God who created you. He is there in the intricate details of who you are. He created you to rise in His glory and to love and be loved. When you see yourself as His daughter and recognize His reflection in you, you will find the end of your rainbow."

Through the windshield, I found the spot where the rainbow ended. It was straight ahead in the middle of the interstate. If I could just keep my eye on it, I would drive right through it. Before I had finished the thought, the carnival of light disappeared. But its beauty stayed with me long after.

❁

# Charming/Chubby

## *Kate Miller*

Charming and chubby. Who says they are mutually exclusive? *Charming* is appealing, pleasant, captivating, magnetic, alluring, and attractive. *Chubby* is seen as decidedly unattractive. For me, chubby means that my body is bigger, that I have love handles, big breasts, a belly. But it does not mean that I am not charming, because charm is a behavior, an attractive personality that exudes happiness and makes people feel better. My big body reflects my big heart under my big breasts and a big laugh in my big belly. My charm comes from my big tendency to savor life at every level and to share it. I cry big tears at sad movies, sad books, or the sorrow in someone else's life. A big smile brightens my face when I see a gorgeous sunset or others' happy moments.

My chubbiness has nothing to do with my charm unless I let my insecurities about being chubby interrupt my charm. When I focus too much on how the world perceives a chubby body, I feel less valuable. My big heart loses capacity to care; my big laugh

**Kate Miller's** *time is spent in school, reading, or listening to music. Having earned a bachelor's degree in English literature, she is now working on a bachelor's degree in psychology with plans to complete a PhD in counseling psychology. Her pets help keep her sane, as does an occasional session of beginner's yoga.*

and smile disappear. The only thing that changes, however, is my focus: I am still chubby, and I can still be charming. But here is the secret, in order for charm to coexist with chubbiness, I have to love my big, chubby body! I have to stop worrying about how the world perceives chubby people because when I pay the world's view no attention, *I am charming.* And when I am charming, no one notices my outer shell, they notice the woman with a big love of life.

# Shame–Less

## Wendy Ulrich

Women have twelve different categories of shame, says Brené Brown in *I Thought It Was Just Me.*[1] Her research suggests that appearance and body image top that list as sources of our shame. I know what you're thinking: "I could have told her this and saved her a lot of research money."

We learn to feel shame about our bodies when parents or friends criticize us (*You've put on a few pounds this summer, haven't you?*). But even when they apply criticism to someone else (*What is she thinking going out like that?*) or to themselves (*I look like a pig!*), we get the message: some body shapes, skin types, hair styles, smells, clothes, facial features, postures, shoe sizes, fingernails, legs, breasts, waists, knees, arms, shoulders, chins, and eyes are *not* acceptable.

It is no exaggeration to say that, as we grow up, women hear and see hundreds of thousands of messages about every aspect

**Wendy Ulrich**, *PhD, is a psychologist and the founder of Sixteen Stones Center for Growth (sixteenstones.net), providing seminar retreats in Utah and Arizona for Latter-day Saint women and their loved ones. Her most recent book is* The Temple Experience: Our Journey toward Holiness *(Springville, UT: Cedar Fort, 2012). She loves knitting, walking, the ocean, family, chocolate, and playing Words with Friends.*

of their physical appearance. And it is not an exaggeration to say that these messages tempt women to feel shame about their inevitable physical imperfections. We can be our own worst enemies: A major source of contention between mothers and daughters is daughters feeling criticized about their appearance.

Many women today are stronger, more health-conscious, and more willing to be seen in public without makeup than those of a generation ago. Yet today's ideals for women are ever more focused on appearance, especially the ability to arouse sexual desire. The sexualization of girls in our culture begins as young as three years old. As I see portrayals of women in the media, I often reflect on our long fight to be treated with equality and respect. I find myself thinking, *We fought the feminist revolution for* this—*to be sex objects for others?* How do we navigate a path toward self-respect and self-definition when sex appeal is our ultimate ideal?

Although *shame* and *guilt* are often used interchangeably, it is helpful to distinguish them. Guilt is a useful feeling of regret about something we have done that violates our moral values or hurts another person. It calls us to empathy for those we have hurt and reminds us to take responsibility, to change, to make amends, to seek reconciliation. Shame, on the other hand, is a destructive sense of humiliation over being flawed, unacceptable, or unworthy when compared to how people "should be." Shame leads us to become defensive, to hide, and to shame others. Feelings of shame lead us to preoccupation with appearances and make us afraid to be too close to others for fear of being judged. Shame makes us prideful when we are successful and insecure when others succeed instead.

Sometimes the very fact that we want to be "virtuous, lovely, or of good report or praiseworthy" (Articles of Faith 1:13) twists us into self-shaming preoccupation with appearing more virtuous and more lovely than others, envying others' good reports, and feeling unworthy unless we merit the praise of the media.

The gospel of Jesus Christ helps heal our shame. It reminds us that our worth is based on our relationship to God, our moral virtues and character, our acts of service and caring—not on living up to the standards of the world. The Savior said, "Blessed are the pure in heart: for they shall see God" (Matthew 5:8). We often think of purity of heart in relation to chastity and virtue. But another aspect of a pure heart is being honest with ourselves about our inherent goodness. When we take ideas about who we are and what is important about us from the media, or from other people instead of from God, we are not being honest with ourselves. Only when we cast those deceits out of our hearts can we have a pure heart, a true basis for valuing ourselves.

Shame does not come from God. Comparisons and judgments based on appearances are not His way of helping us. Not only does God invite us to treat our bodies with reverence, care, and respect, He also teaches women in particular to "lay aside the things of this world, and seek for the things of a better" (Doctrine & Covenants 25:10).

We are created in the image of God. We are beloved by God. We are beholden only to God as our judge. When we deeply trust these truths, the standards of beauty held by the world recede, freeing us to concentrate on what brings joy.

---

NOTE

1. See Brené Brown, *I Thought It Was Just Me (But It Isn't)* (New York: Gotham Publishers, 2007).

❀

# *Beauty in Hot Chocolate*

## *Jessica Larsen*

I thought I became beautiful the summer I turned thirteen. That was the summer *The Princess Diaries* came out and, along with Mia Thermopolis, I tossed my glasses, cut my hair, and rustled up a new wardrobe. But insecurities aren't thrown out as easily as worn-out jeans, and I soon discovered I was still pursuing somebody else's idea of beauty.

For years afterward, I defined myself by relationships—I was a sister, a friend, a daughter, even a girlfriend. I loved these roles and the people I spent time with, but happiness seemed evasive, temperamental. After too many months of hiding and crying in corners (wearing waterproof mascara, naturally), I pretended I was a heroine in a chick flick, enrolled in the BYU London study abroad program, and booked a flight to England.

My first week was a disaster. I spent the first days desperately trying to latch on to other students who seemed to know what they were doing. The result? I saw plays I didn't like, galleries I didn't appreciate, and ended up wishing for a good witch or a pair

---

**Jessica Larsen** *is a native Californian who enjoys road trips, cheap pizza, and Audrey Hepburn films. She is a freelance writer and editor, specializing in children's literature. Jessica currently lives with her husband and laptop in Arizona.*

of red shoes to take me back home where I belonged. Yet all that changed one Saturday afternoon when the rain hung indecisively between the sky and the pavement in a heavy fog.

That was the Saturday I set off through Kensington in search of adventure with only my journal and pen for company. No more laughing or crying on cue like an audience in an old TV studio, I told myself. Today I get to do just what *I* want to do. Today I find out what *I* like. I promised myself I'd stop at the first place that caught my eye.

Three streets later, I saw them—a coffee shop and a bookstore leaning into each other like sisters telling secrets. This was not one of the *haute culture* places my London friends preferred; the coffee shop seemed a little shabby, but comfortable. *I'd like to be that comfortable with myself,* I thought, and ducked inside.

I sat in the corner (my friends always preferred to sit in the middle) and felt at home. When I got my cocoa, the cup was large enough to wrap both hands around, and the thick, whipped cream curled up over the brim. I took a sip, and hot liquid eased down my throat and warmed me like a hug.

It isn't just the drink, I decided as I wrote in my journal. I'm learning that I like London hot chocolate better than Starbucks, but I'm also learning I like being with myself. I'm in London, but I'm not at the newest play or the hippest pub—and that's okay. I'm doing exactly what I want to do, and that's enough.

That was the beginning of my journey to true beauty. It wasn't a big day (honestly, blowing it up this big makes me feel like I'm trying to be Virginia Woolf or something), but it was the start of self-definition and independence from others' ideals. So much has happened since then—I found the courage to serve a Mormon mission and to graduate from college—but I still continue to grow. I still redefine myself. And if life gets too busy, I simply duck into a coffee shop and enjoy a cup of hot chocolate with myself.

# *Beauty Lost*

## Lisa Tensmeyer Hansen

My third-grade teacher turned me into a math lover. While I waited for one of the many things third-graders wait for (lunch, recess, going home) she would take a sheet of lined elementary school paper and write an "N problem" in red ballpoint pen. Then she'd walk by my chair and slip it onto my desk. I would tune out the world until that "N" was defined. When I'd give it back to her, she'd take almost no time to pen another. I don't know how many problems she gave me that school year, but I remember being happy she filled my empty time with fascinating equations.

Third grade was a hard year in other ways. Boys. Clothes. I couldn't figure these out. A pretty wrapped package in my desk turned out to be deodorant. People who didn't play by rules often won the games, and one girl who studied spelling more than anyone else always seemed to get the lowest grade, which was posted every Friday. She and I decided to study together one week

**Lisa Tensmeyer Hansen** *finished raising seven children and is having a hard time sitting still. A doctoral candidate at Brigham Young University in marriage and family therapy, she is a managing editor of the* BYU Women's Studies Journal, *serves on the board of local arts organizations, writes music with her husband, and walks every morning with her BFF.*

until she could spell every word. Then during the test, I borrowed her eraser every time a word was announced and surreptitiously pointed out changes she needed to make. I'm sure I borrowed her eraser ten times during that little test, but my teacher (sitting three feet away and watching us during the ordeal) never said a word, even when my classmate's score topped the list. Our silent confederacy in pursuit of this girl's vision of herself as a good student still touches me. Somehow my teacher correctly guessed I would never cheat again.

Third grade didn't last forever, and I went on to trust my instincts, and to enjoy math—a lot. And I think I have my teacher to thank for both those gifts. So when I take out my third-grade class photo, I look at her picture with fondness.

No, wait—I don't. And I'm sad about that.

The day we got our third-grade class pictures was a big one. We waited for months for the day when we'd walk into our classroom and discover on our desks, like Christmas surprises, big white envelopes with our faces shining through the clear plastic. After we each pulled them out and made our assessments of each other's triumph in the picture-taking arena, our teacher sat us down. She asked each of us to take out our class picture and lay it on our desks. She was very sorry, she told us, but she did not want a picture of herself in our class photo. She didn't like the way she looked. She said she would come around with scissors and ask our permission to carefully cut her picture out of every one of them. Which she did.

I remember not understanding this. As she worked her scissors to get the edges just right to excise herself from my photo, I felt something else slip away. I think it was confidence that what was inside me was what really mattered.

My teacher's compassionate heart was truly beautiful. I have no doubt I would still see that beauty if I had her picture. I would love to see her face again—the beautiful face of inspiration.

# My Butterfly Journey

## Name Withheld

Beauty is all around me—in the waves of the Pacific, the sky from here to the horizon, the sand where I sit with the women in my family, my mother's confidence, and my eighty-year-old grandmother's contentment. But I forget sometimes that my spirit is as beautiful as all that. As a ten-year-old, I saw myself as chubby, thought I had a weird nose, and believed I didn't have a pretty smile. "Why can't I look like that girl?" I would ask.

My mother has been an angel in my life. I've looked up to her as my hero. Instead of chiding me for my lack of confidence, my mother came into my room every night to tell me she loves me, listing the ways I am beautiful to her. She gave me the nickname "butterfly," which I accepted gladly. Her daily ministrations worked magic in me until I found my way out of my cocoon.

# Truth Beautiful

## Elaine Rumsey Wagner

I remember sitting in my grandmother's kitchen
Surrounded by the warmth of the wood furnace,
   stoked hot
Against the four-foot drifts of the Snake River plain.
She told me how beautiful I was,
Her creased hands against my cheeks.
She talked about the beauty of youth that doesn't need
Lipstick and cream blushers.
Her hands, part of the early morning crew that cut
   potatoes at spring planting,
Pulled the brown dirt fruit of Idaho
Across the knife edge in front of her,
Shining wet in the dimness of the spud pit.
With such fruit, she had
Piled dollar after dollar

**Elaine Rumsey Wagner** *has a bachelor's in math from Brigham Young University and a master's in mathematics from California State University, Fresno. She has four sons, one daughter, one wonderful husband, two ridiculous dogs, and two fluffy cats. She lives in Rexburg, where she teaches math at BYU–Idaho, juggles schedules, shovels in the winter, mows in the summer, and in her spare time (four to six A.M.), she writes.*

Into her sons' college accounts
To make my father's life, and then mine.
She excelled at Latin
Before she had to quit school.
I wondered if it had done her any good.
I thought she didn't really understand
Me, mourning my small-town lack of boyfriend.
Now I know more.
I walk in the sun of California
To teach my junior college math class
My students ask,
When are we ever going to use this?
I look out at a sea of youth
And I see beauty.
Sometimes they lose it in the trying,
Clothes tight and short, teetering on four-inch heels,
Pierced, tattooed, smoking, posing,
But in their eyes, a longing
For someone to tell them
They are Beautiful.
I visited my grandmother last, after her stroke,
In the Idaho nursing home next to the Snake,
Past the gray ice chunks in the parking lot.
In her wheelchair, hands constantly shaking, she smiled
As my sisters and I sang Christmas songs.
She knew me, which was rare.
Her too-frail hand on my arm,
She asked me to take her with me.
Then she told me I was Beautiful,
So Beautiful.

# Beauty—A Divine Gift

## Rachel Uda Murdock

*Will not wear glasses because of vanity.*

That's what my doctor wrote in my medical records when I was six years old. *Has anorexic tendencies,* he said when I was twelve. Indeed. My teenage years were filled with constant anxiety about what I looked like. I could never get my hair to do anything flattering, I had problems with acne, my clothes weren't cool, and I worried every day about getting fat.

Dating taught me plenty. If a boy liked me, I must be pretty. If he broke up with me, I was ugly, fat, and worthless.

At twenty, I was ninety-five pounds and full-blown anorexic. My collar and rib bones jutted sharply but it didn't matter. I just couldn't eat.

My parents hospitalized me and when I was released, I entered an out-treatment program. The counseling was grueling but helped. Gradually I gained control of the urge not to eat. I still wasn't happy with how I looked, but the eating disorder and I

**Rachel Uda Murdock** *lives in Hawaii with her husband and three children. They own and manage a vacation rental management and cleaning company. She enjoys politics, entrepreneurship, music, blogging, and Hawaiian sunsets.*

called a truce. It never took over my life again. But my basic belief that I was ugly, unlovable, and unworthy remained.

Shortly thereafter, I served a mission in Japan. I grew in many ways and gained forty pounds. I was disgusted by my appearance but dealt with it by focusing on the work. In Japanese culture, it isn't rude to tell someone they are fat, and on several occasions people told me how fat I'd become. The comments hurt, but I pushed them into the place I stored proof that I was ugly and kept working.

After returning home from my mission, I met a wonderful, caring, and compassionate man. He saw me as beautiful inside and out, and it was easy to fall in love with him. Getting married helped take the pressure off my wounded self-image. Still, on occasion, if my husband was upset or we had a disagreement, I immediately attributed it to the fact that I wasn't beautiful enough and was hopelessly unlovable.

We had two children when I was diagnosed with cancer. I was twenty-eight years old. My first question to the doctor was, "Am I going to lose my hair?" Never mind that I had cancer, that there was a large tumor growing in my chest, and that I would die without treatment. . . . I was going to lose my hair! I was going to be bald!

I began treatment, which consisted of toxic chemotherapy cocktails being injected into a port in my chest every week. A month later, my hair began falling out. It was traumatic to lose large clumps of long hair, so I cut it short, then finally asked my husband to shave my head.

I cried as he shaved it, but by the time he was done, I was resigned. I went to look in the mirror and as I ran my fingers over my head I reminded myself there was nothing I could do about it.

As I got sicker, my eyebrows began thinning and the steroids made me gain weight. I started avoiding mirrors all together. I was a troll. I was the hairless Gollum from *Lord of the Rings*.

My energy level dropped dramatically. I couldn't drive because of the medications I was taking, and I occasionally had to use a wheelchair. I couldn't even hold my children. My mother moved in to take care of us so my husband could keep working. I was completely dependent on her help.

During treatment, I also had surgery to remove my gallbladder. By the end of the two-week hospital stay, I noticed there were some stray hairs growing like weeds out of my head. Frustrated, I took thick pieces of medical tape and stuck them to my head, then with quick yanks ripped them off. When I saw what I had done, I began to panic. There was so much hair on the tape. I didn't know I still had that much—and I had just ripped it all out!

In tears, I began to pray. I was completely and utterly humbled. I was at the mercy of God and with my bald head lowered in prayer, I found myself willing to accept anything He had to offer. What He gave me in that moment surprised me. I was suddenly filled with warmth and peace. I felt His love envelop me. I realized in that moment that I was more valuable to Him than I could imagine. As weak and helpless as I was, I knew that I was a divine child of God.

It was an extraordinary feeling. No longer could I deny that I was lovable. I couldn't even deny that I was beautiful. God made me, and He made me beautiful. I had been beautiful all along but had never acknowledged it. Looking in the mirror at my puffy, eyebrow-less face, dark-grooved circles under my eyes, and my shiny Gollum head, I was a beautiful child of God. Why had I never realized this before?

It was because of my pride. Alma taught the Zoramites: "And now, because ye are compelled to be humble blessed are ye; for a man sometimes, if he is compelled to be humble, seeketh repentance; and now surely, whosoever repenteth shall find mercy" (Alma 32:13).

Is it a sin to have low self-esteem? I would have to say yes. It is a sin of ingratitude. The lack of esteem for one's self comes from despair. Moroni taught that "despair cometh because of iniquity" (Moroni 10:22).

Medical and psychological theories try to explain why girls become anorexic. Perhaps the tendency is in their genes or they learn to process social dynamics in self-defeating ways. And of course, there are horribly unrealistic images in the media to teach them to be dissatisfied with themselves. But what I came to realize is that my self-loathing was actually related to ingratitude for the body given to me by Heavenly Father. I had chosen to believe the cruel lies of the devil, who was so jealous of the body I had been given he was determined to make me hate it, and then destroy it. I had given in to the enticings of the world, being consumed with my outward appearance, giving in to the natural man. King Benjamin taught:

"For the natural man is an enemy to God, and has been from the fall of Adam, and will be, forever and ever, unless he yields to the enticings of the Holy Spirit, and putteth off the natural man and becometh a saint through the atonement of Christ the Lord, and becometh as a child, submissive, meek, humble, patient, full of love, willing to submit to all things which the Lord seeth fit to inflict upon him, even as a child doth submit to his father" (Mosiah 3:19).

I was ready to put off the natural (wo)man. As long as I could continue to feel that sweet and peaceful love from my Heavenly Father, I was ready to submit to whatever He saw fit to "inflict" upon me. I would get through this experience with beauty, patience, and faith. I would not despair.

I had been stripped of my crown of hair; now I was puffed up like a marshmallow, and without energy, it hardly seemed sometimes that I had a life to be grateful for. But I had stopped believing lies and started realizing how much God loves me.

I do not believe Heavenly Father gave me cancer to punish me for not knowing more about Him. Bad things just happen in this life. That's how we are tested. But because all things work together for our good, I will be forever grateful that through that terrible experience, I learned to feel God's love for me more abundantly.

# The Beauty underneath the Surface

## S. Michael Wilcox

A few years ago I had an opportunity to take a tour group to the Middle East. We stopped at the Red Sea on the Egyptian-Israeli border. It is a desolate, dry, barren place. I could not see anything green for miles. When we drove across the border, I remember looking around and seeing nothing but rock and sky—nothing seemed to live there. I thought, as I surveyed the dry, desolate scenery, "Whomever God assigned to create this part of his world needs to go back and take Creation 101 again, because they didn't do a very good job here."

Later that day, I put on a snorkel mask and swam just a few feet off the coast to look at the coral reefs. In some places the reef lies just a few inches under the surface of the water. What a different world that was! Beautiful corals of every color, fish of all varieties displaying the most wonderful patterns. Here was life at its fullest! There are few places I have been where one can

**S. Michael Wilcox** *received his PhD from the University of Colorado and recently retired after thirty-seven years as an institute instructor for the Church Educational System. A popular speaker and award-winning author, his previous publications include* House of Glory, Walking on Water, *and* 10 Great Souls I Want to Meet in Heaven.

see more beautiful life than snorkeling in the Red Sea. As I was looking at all that magnificent splendor, I remembered my first judgment of the area. I had condemned this part of the earth's surface as a godforsaken place. As I swam along the surface of the water with my eyes peering into the depths, I could feel God's smile and his laugh—I'm sure he has a delightful laugh. I was enjoying the wonder of his creation which had been hidden from my view by just a few inches of water. When the impression was sufficiently deep, the Lord whispered to me, "Michael, you must learn to see all things, and all places, and all people, as you have learned to see today." God always sees the beauty underneath the surface!

❀

# Mother, Grandmother, Sisters, Daughters, Me: Us

## Laura Craner

Mother.

As she sits in front of her vanity with the afternoon sun slanting through the French doors and across her face, I surprise her. A small, Avon pink faux tortoiseshell case is on the counter. The tweezers are in hand. One eyebrow is arched. Her face is half-turned toward me, half toward the many-bulbed mirror. A drawer full of creams and lotions and powders and colors is fully opened. Her posture is straight. Her neck is extended. Her dark eyes are unblinking.

Her expression: Do you need something?

I feel as if I should feel uncomfortable—as if I am interrupting something grown-up, something secret, something powerful—but I am not uncomfortable. Maybe this is what I need.

She never likes to be photographed, but I sneak as many pictures as possible because no matter what, Mother is beautiful.

---

**Laura Hilton Craner** *is a mommy and sometimes writer. She lives (and writes) in Colorado with four children. She is a writer and editor for an online content and marketing company and occasionally blogs at the Mormon Arts and Culture website* A Motley Vision *(www.motleyvision.org). When she isn't reading, writing, or cleaning up after someone, Laura spends her time hiking, canning, and dabbling in the expressive arts.*

• • •

Grandmother.

Lying in the hospital bed, she is tenuously posed on her side by the hospice staff, her fingers threading through the bars. At first sight, I am struck by her appearance: long fingernails slightly yellowed and glittery from week-old nail polish; hair that was previously coiffed and permed close to the head now a shock of smooth white standing out from her pale pink scalp. Her eyelids flutter open. She spots the red roses on the bedside table.

Her words: "What are those? They're beautiful."

I tell her they are roses and that they are for her. She stares with deep blue childlike eyes. In her advanced dementia everything is new. She turns her eyes to me and quizzically asks who I am. Before I can answer she tells me I am beautiful. Her gaze shifts to the ceiling and she gasps in wonder. "Beautiful," she breathes. "Simply beautiful."

As she dies, she is seeing things the rest of us cannot. She is beautiful.

• • •

Sisters.

There are four of us. Older: Snow White, with pale skin, red lips, and raven hair. Dramatic and striving. Younger: Sleeping Beauty, except she is shades of caramel and chocolate instead of blonde and blue-eyed. Young and dreaming. Middle: Belle, with my nose in a book and mousy hair in a ponytail. Restless and wondering. Youngest: Died in infancy; there are no fairy tales about that. We could just as easily be: Older, Charlotte Bronte. Younger, Jane Austen. Middle, Emily Dickinson. Youngest, lost in translation. A canon of femininity, we are each other's truest mirrors and most frustrating distortions.

Our question: With you and without you, how am I myself?

Looking at them, looking at me, looking at each other, we define ourselves by what *she* is and what *I* am not. We are finding beautiful.

●  ●  ●

Daughters.

Three of them. Oldest, eight years old. Standing in front of a mirror swishing a white dress back and forth. Fingers caressing the beads and silk. Lingering barefoot on the dressing room floor, she can't get enough of seeing herself. The eyes of her reflection meet mine and sparkle. Middle, six years old. Running on a soccer field, the tip of her tongue sticking out with concentration. Chasing the ball. Catching it. Kicking it in the goal. She wants to make sure I am watching. Youngest, seventeen months old. Standing. Wobbling. Steadying. Lifting one little foot centimeters off the ground and placing it barely in front of the other. Then lifting the other foot centimeters off the ground and placing it a step forward. Finally walking. She giggles with arms outstretched and looks me in the eye, knowing I'm there.

Each of them asking: *Do you see me?*

Through motherly lenses made up of both rose-colored glasses and adult eyes of worry, I cannot see them enough. They are achingly beautiful.

●  ●  ●

Me.

Almost thirty, married ten years, mother of four. I'm shorter than I'd hoped, much more freckled than I remember, and stretch-marked from belly button to upper thigh. Breasts that swelled when I was on the pill now droop. My hands are worn from housework. I usually don't recognize myself in the mirror. This wasn't my plan. I am both younger and older than I ever thought I'd be. So young to be married so long with so many kids. So old compared to my contemporaries, who are just now getting married and having children.

My question: What have I become?

I have traded self-indulgence for sacrifice, convention for fulfillment, comfort for strength. Realizing beauty is not tethered to youth is what it means to be a woman.

•   •   •

Mother, grandmother, sisters, daughters, me: Us.
We are beautiful.

# Why I Don't Hide My Freckles Anymore: Rescuing Inner Beauty

## Lisa Rumsey Harris

I believe passionately in the kind of beauty that springs from the unexpected. But when it comes to beauty in my own life, I'm uncomfortable. Couldn't we talk about shoes instead?

No? But yesterday I found a gorgeous pair of suede cheetah heels, 50 percent off! Okay. Back to beauty. Here's why I get uncomfortable. The world's idea of beauty is just plain painful. It relies on *perfection* and *judgment*. Let's start with perfection. Society thinks beauty is to be without flaw. And I know I have flaws. So I run from beauty. Because someday soon, someone will discover what really lurks beneath the Spanx and spray tan. (Side note: What do you get when a woman takes off her Spanx? *A flabalanche!*) Advertisers convince us they have a product that will make us perfect, disguise our defects, and create an invincible facade. Were you born with stumpy lashes? Eyelash extensions!

**Lisa Rumsey Harris** *grew up writing stories and riding horses in southeastern Idaho. She received bachelor's and master's degrees in English from Brigham Young University, where she now teaches honors and advanced writing classes. Lisa lives in Orem, Utah, with her husband, Griffin, and her two adorable daughters. Her new book,* The Unlikely Gift of Treasure Blume, *was released in November 2012.*

Plagued with acne? Buy our cream! Short legs? Tall shoes! Too tall? Flat shoes! (It really does all come back to shoes.)

I have run from beauty most of my life. See, I have freckles. And no amount of my mother's claiming that they were "kisses from the sun" made them less objectionable. As a kid, I tried to scrape them off with a butter knife. As a preteen, I counted down the days until Mom would let me wear makeup so I could cover them. Under a thick layer of foundation and powder, I felt safer. Hiding worked pretty well until I hit college.

During my freshman year, I worked at the Sundance stables as a trail guide. Part of my responsibility was to muck out thirty stalls twice a day. So when I came home at night, you could smell me before you could see me. And when you saw me, chances were my hair would be cowboy-hat-crushed and I'd be sporting a dirt mustache. Any vestige of makeup would have been eroded by dust, sun, and sweat. I arrived at my apartment in just this state one night to find my roommates gathered with our family home evening brothers. One of the guys (a rich kid from California who drove a Land Rover) shot me a look. He panned all the way up me, then down my other side. He had flirted with me a couple of times, but I could tell this was not a flirty look. "You don't have any makeup on!" he shouted. "Your skin is blindingly white. And you have freckles!" He got up and left the room. Apparently he thought I'd lied to him about being attractive. From that point on, there was no "love at home" in our fake family.

That painful memory brings me to the second nerve-wracking component of beauty: judgment. You know the old adage: "Beauty is in the eye of the beholder." Never mind if the beholder is a shallow, conceited jerk who happens to drive a Land Rover. He still gets to judge because he's the beholder. Now that's unfair.

Another story to illustrate: My mom was at Costco after

getting her hair done. As she and my dad sat at a table eating hot dogs, an elderly lady (eighty-five-plus) whom Mom didn't know approached her and exclaimed, "You're beautiful!" My mom murmured a quiet thank-you. But the lady didn't stop there. Instead she shouted: "Hey folks, look at this beautiful woman!" The people in the food court didn't know how to react. One guy dropped his pizza. "Don't you see this beautiful woman?" the lady persisted, pointing at my mother. The food court answered with embarrassed silence. Mom wanted to crawl under the table along with the guy's pizza. The lady finally moved on, but Mom said she could feel everyone in the food court looking at her. She felt like a pig at a country fair, with every onlooker sizing up her merits. She wanted to shout "Hey, I know I'm old." Instead she grabbed her hot dog and ran as fast as she could. Just thinking about that episode still makes her cringe. Now you should know, in reading this story, that my mother is beautiful. She truly is. And yet, being on display like that embarrassed her deeply. It's the idea that we're on display for judgment that makes us doubt, makes us want to duck, makes us shrug and shiver. It does me. How about you? Wish we were talking about shoes yet?

But what if perfection and judgment weren't what beauty was about? And what if we didn't need the world's permission to enjoy our own Beauty? Recapturing *that*? Now that's more exciting to me than shoes.

Here is the truth (and John Keats knew it): "'Beauty is truth, truth beauty,'—that is all."[1] His words resonate with me. True beauty is the core of a person: the essence. True beauty is born of resilience and individuality. It says: *You are intrinsically of worth and value, no matter what you look like.* That idea gives me strength.

At this point, you may be thinking, "Inner beauty? Really?"

I know where you're coming from. *Inner beauty* is a cliché

that causes eye-rolling. Some people even use it as a code phrase for "not-so-good-looking." If you ever find a man who compliments you on your inner beauty, the saying goes, you should probably run. But even if the words are tired, the idea remains. *Inner beauty* is *inner truth*. Truth is beautiful.

Gerard Manley Hopkins called the distinctive pattern and individuality inside each of us *inscape*.[2] Our inscape bears the mark of our divine creator, inviting us to commune with Him. Our inscape is beautiful.

I think of *inscape* when I'm in the temple (the only place I can count on consistently feeling beautiful). Everyone is beautiful there: young and old, married, single, short, tall, wide, or slim. Beauty there does not require a flawless body or face. The temple is awash with beauty, lit by divine light. When I'm there, I'm part of that beauty and I can see by that light. We are God's creations, and His beauty comes alive in us there.

Even outside the temple, the faces I find beautiful have flaws. I see beauty in my mother's silver hair, in the gap-toothed grin of my six-year-old. I see beauty in the exhausted eyes of my students at midterms. I see it when I face the young women in my ward every week and together we repeat the words "We are daughters of our Heavenly Father who loves us, and we love Him."[3]

It takes courage to look at ourselves, sharing the hyperawareness of our own imperfections and flaws, and then say that we are beautiful. But when we do that, a funny thing happens. We start to believe it. We are empowered to see beauty in ourselves, and that leads to finding beauty in the people around us. And then, surprise! We find beauty in the strength of our own imperfect bodies, in the mysterious swirl of fingerprints left on the wall by a mischievous finger painter, in the way a grandmother's eyes crinkle in the corners when she laughs. Not flawless, but real and true and individual.

Today, I'm comfortable in my own blindingly white skin. I've embraced my freckles, thanks to Gerard Manley Hopkins. Not only did he teach me about *inscape,* but he also wrote a poem called "Pied Beauty" that praises all dappled things:

> All things counter, original, spare, strange;
> Whatever is fickle, freckled (who knows how?)
> With swift, slow; sweet, sour; adazzle, dim;
> He fathers-forth whose beauty is past change:
>     Praise him.[4]

So I stopped hating my freckles. I married a man who loves them, and loves me. I smile when I see freckles sprinkled across the bridge of my daughter's nose. I tell her they are kisses from the sun. I don't hide mine under layers of makeup anymore. The freckles are part of me: a quirky, individual, distinct part of me— much like my love of shoes. I'm wearing the cheetah heels on Sunday with a red dress. And I've decided freckles are beautiful.

---

## NOTES

1. John Keats, "Ode on a Grecian Urn," in *Ode on a Grecian Urn, The Eve of St. Agnes: And Other Poems* (Boston: Houghton Mifflin, 1898), 14.

2. See Stephen Greenblatt, et. al., eds. "Gerard Manley Hopkins," in *Norton Anthology of English Literature*, 8th ed., vol. 2 (New York: W. W. Norton, 2006), 2159.

3. LDS Young Women theme; available at https://www.lds.org/young -women/personal-progress/young-women-theme?lang=eng; accessed 25 July 2013.

4. Gerard Manley Hopkins, "Pied Beauty," in *Literature: An Introduction to Fiction, Poetry, and Drama*, 4th ed., X. J. Kennedy, ed. (Boston: Little, Brown and Company, 1987), 485.

# On Beauty: Coming to Terms

### Susan Chieko Eliason

*Look to your roots, in order to reclaim your future.*
—Ghanaian proverb

Among my very first memories is gazing with admiration at my beautiful mother while she was getting ready to go out with my dad. I remember one night in particular when they were getting dressed for a Gold and Green Ball. Dad looked smashing in his dark suit and tie—to this day he remains the most handsome man I've ever seen in or out of Hollywood—but my *mama* that night. Oh my.

She swished past me in her sleek taffeta gown, clip-on gold earrings dangling. Somehow the cuddly, peanut butter-smudged matron in a pink housecoat had become a bona fide glamour queen. I loved the way she smoothed crimson lipstick over her lips (and cheeks!) and piled her shiny hair up high. Glancing

---

**Susan Chieko Eliason** *is a consultant at Brigham Young University's Center for Teaching and Learning, assigned to work primarily with faculty at the Marriott School of Management and the School of Religious Education. Susan has lived and traveled with her family throughout the world, finding her greatest delights in missionary work and studying the languages of her host countries.*

down occasionally at me, her shameless admirer, she murmured, "When you grow bigger, you can dress up just like me!" My heart danced at the thought, and I made note of that glorious promise. Meanwhile, I borrowed her high heels and toddled around the house or smeared color on my cheeks as often as she allowed.

Fast-forward several decades to the present. I smile at a picture of my mother as she is now. I see the same warm smile, glowing skin, beckoning eyes. Alas, the chestnut mane has been replaced by thinning white hair, and my father is too diplomatic (and smart) to point out that he observes about fifty pounds there he didn't marry. But Mother remains the epitome of beauty. As she stood in front of a theater one day—white hair, cane, and all—a car paused at the curb beside her and the driver remarked, "You are the most beautiful lady I've ever seen." Little children tell her the same thing all the time at grocery stores and at church. Grumpy old men and neighborhood bullies melt when she walks by.

From my middle-aged (and arguably more objective) point of view, I'd say she's even more beautiful than she was in her younger years. Her eyes now shine through a lifetime of challenges triumphantly overcome—retina and cataract surgeries, for starters, but also some generous servings of illness, disappointment, and betrayal. One hip and two knee replacements bear witness to the toll of decades of dedicated caregiving, including lengthy ministrations to both of her parents and to my father.

I told my mother recently that she is remarkably attractive and *attracting* to all who know her because she has learned to harness the most powerful force in the universe: Love. Should you happen to look up "Susan's mother" in the dictionary, you would see, simply, *Love.* Verb, noun, adjective *lovely,* adverb *lovingly*—the only word needed to tell the entire story in her Book of Life.

A few months ago I received an invitation to write an essay on whether I'd made peace with beauty in my life. Had I come to terms with my physical imperfections? Oh, the multiple false starts and torn pages that followed. I could write an entire book, for example, on my eventual discovery that life doesn't have to be one long, miserable diet. I'm learning to love my body and feed it only what it needs. This means learning to deal with the stresses of life in ways other than chocolate chips and ice cream.

Another side trip in writing about my quest to make peace with beauty included reflections on five years as a stake Relief Society president at Brigham Young University. My service included helping young college women struggling with eating disorders, life-planning issues, and general angst. "Looking great," of course, was (and remains) high on the priority list for that demographic. And it's a worthy pursuit—"as far as it is translated correctly." Destructive outcomes often follow the excessive pursuit of society's beauty standards.

Yet another attempt to write a piece on beauty featured an incident I witnessed in a women's restroom. The occasion was a singles' conference, and as I was washing my hands, a woman next to me gave herself the once-over in the full-length mirror, tossed her head, and declared under her breath, "Just one more day before this shindig's over—I gotta make it count!" I felt the urgency of her hope. When our opportunities are circumscribed by what we see in the mirror, we all suffer.

Then, suddenly, it happens: I remember with perfect clarity that magical evening long ago when my mama was dressing up for the ball. Her allure was spellbinding to her four-year-old and, I suspect, to everyone else she encountered that night. I speed up the memory train a moment later and reflect on more recent observations. Now, in the full bloom of age, Mother's beauty is softly striking and almost indefinable; an illumination from within bespeaks victory in her experience of mortality. And just the same as all those years ago when I watched her preparing for her big night out, I still want to be just like her someday.

Yes, I think I've finally figured out the beauty thing. I've long since worn my own high heels, but I hope with all my heart eventually to blossom in the footsteps of my mother.

❁

# Once Upon a Time—A Tale of Beauty and Strength

### Ronald Bartholomew

I grew up in Lehi, Utah, back when it was a small town. It didn't take long for me to realize I didn't have a whole lot of social currency in my neighborhood. In our small farming community it seemed the only thing that mattered for a young man was physical strength and athleticism. After spending six elementary school years playing by myself during recess or being picked last on all the teams, I finally left that lonely experience and started junior high, a place that was intimidating to me on multiple levels. The antiquated school building had no lockers, but had coat hooks instead, which were placed just high enough off the floor to enable the larger boys the opportunity of "hanging up" the smaller ones and leaving them there until someone came along to rescue them!

My mother, who typically remembers things in more-than-glowing reality, has often recalled that the only thing she

---

**Ronald Bartholomew** *has been a religion instructor for twenty-eight years. He is currently teaching at the institute of religion adjacent to Utah Valley University, and he has taught in the religion departments at Brigham Young University (Provo), the BYU Salt Lake Center, and BYU–Idaho. He and his wife, Kirsten, are the parents of seven children and have four grandchildren. He is an avid bicycle commuter.*

remembers about me during these years was how many times I came home from school black-eyed and bloody-nosed. The same young men who delighted in hanging me from those coat hooks also took great delight in chasing me home from school and pounding the daylights out of me. My body size made me an easy target.

As I entered high school, I was horrified to discover that the lockers I had yearned for in junior high were simply my next nightmare—the bigger boys demonstrated that I fit perfectly. If I ever design lockers, I'm going to put a release button on the inside! It was during one locker episode I decided on a plan. If I could make the high school football team (or any team, for that matter), I might earn some respect. Just maybe those looming man-menaces might end up defending me on the field! The coach, however, took one look at me and shook his head. I tried out for team after team, and the coach (who was also the coach of all the other teams) rejected my efforts. Not one team let me play. I needed a new survival plan.

Then it happened. At the height of my sports failures, I was approached by the cheerleading squad. They explained to me that they were nominating me for student-body president and they wanted to run my campaign. My jaw dropped. They went on. They had been watching me, they said, and they were sure I would do a better job than the popular, handsome, athletic young man who would be running against me. I couldn't believe it. At first I suspected a trick (and so did some of my teachers). But the girls' sincerity eventually won me over and I found myself taking a closer look at what they were saying. Being a popular sports star might not be everything after all. They seemed to want a leader who was energetic and hopeful, even if he wasn't always successful. They wanted someone who would listen to them, someone who would take them seriously. They wanted someone who knew how to pick himself up and keep on going. They wanted someone who had experience on the less-arrogant side of life.

Much to my shock, and everybody else's too, I not only won the race, I won by a landslide. As a boy who thought his lack of social currency rested on his physical limitations, I had to rethink life. Here's what I decided: Life is not a beauty contest. The human spirit needs more than beauty and strength.

Sometime during that year, the cross-country team recruited me too. (They didn't have a coach to discourage them from asking me.) What I discovered was that being chased home every day from school had developed my legs, heart, and lungs for long-distance running! Even with all that preparation, I still wasn't great. At the end of our final meet, the two fastest young men on our team (who had already crossed the finish line), ran the course backwards to find me. I'll never forget what they did then. They flanked me on both sides and with kind words of encouragement ran with me to the finish line. The human spirit definitely needs more than beauty and strength. We are all in this together, and we need each other. That is the real beauty and strength of life.

# Beauty Evolution

## Linda Flores

I was born in China but moved to the ethnically diverse area of Seattle when I was eight years old. I didn't realize I looked different from other people until I started practicing makeup. I was confused about why I wasn't able to recreate the *right* look on my almond-shaped eyes. It was discouraging to imagine I would never look like the models I saw in magazines.

Despite this letdown, I kept thinking about an inspiring quote. The first chapter of *Bobbi Brown Beauty Evolution: A Guide to a Lifetime of Beauty* taught me, "Beauty is feeling good without having to look in the mirror." Somehow this reminded me that I could feel beautiful without conforming to the media's definition of beauty.

I started exercising frequently, which helped me feel great. I signed up for gymnastics and learned to appreciate my strong and healthy body. Later I joined choir and the ballroom dance team,

**Linda Flores** *is the embodiment of multiculturalism. She is a Chinese-American woman with a Hispanic name, a heavily Pacific Islander–influenced upbringing, a passion for Latin dancing, and a deep interest in African American studies (as well as all cultures). Her goal in life is to inspire and assist others in reaching their goals and fulfilling their potential.*

which further improved my self-image. I also enjoyed playing piano and earning good grades because I found out I was good at both. As I improved myself, I grew to like myself more, even though I still believed I wasn't as pretty as the other girls in my school.

Another inspiring quote stayed with me. In the movie *Mr. Skeffington*, Bette Davis says, "A woman's beautiful only when she is loved."[1] At first look, I found this quote a bit disturbing, because it implied that a woman's attractiveness depends on someone else's affection. But on second thought, this quote encouraged me to develop positive attributes like kindness, selflessness, and cheerfulness that make me more beautiful inside and out. Still, when I moved away from home for the first time, I found out Bette Davis was right. By surrounding myself with people who loved me, it was easier to see my own beauty.

I am especially touched that the Lord would respond directly to my insecurities about being beautiful. I was baptized into the LDS Church on my eighteenth birthday and received my patriarchal blessing shortly thereafter. I was surprised to see the word *beautiful* mentioned nine times in my blessing. The Lord seemed to want to reassure me, telling me how beautiful I was, how much more beautiful I would become, and even how to *be* beautiful—by being cultured and enjoying the works of good men and women.

I have found this counsel to be true. I feel my senses awaken and my spirit enliven after attending a concert of well-performed music, reading an eloquent piece of prose, dancing with a good partner to uplifting songs, and enjoying other cultural activities. As I follow the counsel in my blessing, I do, in fact, feel beautiful without looking in the mirror.

---

NOTE

1. Julius J. Epstein and Philip G. Epstein (screenwriters), *Mr. Skeffington* (Hollywood: Warner Brothers, 1944).

# Thank You, Body

## Anna Packard

Thank you *body* for allowing me to experience every day completely.

Thank you *eyes* for the opportunity to see the beauty and majesty of the world around me.

Thank you *nose* for the pleasure of smelling delicious food and the familiar smell of my husband.

Thank you *lips* for tender moments kissing the soft doughy skin of my newborn daughter.

Thank you *mouth* for allowing me to nourish myself with food and to enjoy new tastes.

Thank you *tongue* for allowing me to transform my thoughts and feelings into words I can share with others through conversation, laughter, and song.

Thank you *brain* . . . for everything—for the memories you encode, for the emotions you allow me to feel, for the deep

---

**Anna Packard** *is a licensed clinical psychologist who is passionate about women's issues. She works mainly with women struggling with eating disorders and loves every minute of it. She is mother to two animated daughters and a sweet angel son in heaven and strives to embrace the lessons life has to offer. To honor her body and herself, Anna eats chocolate every day, drinks lots of water, exercises, and pauses each evening to watch the sunset.*

thoughts you allow me to generate, for the information you allow me to store and analyze, for allowing me to integrate my experiences into a cohesive sense of self.

Thank you *lungs* for allowing me to breathe *in* the richness of life—the bitter cold in the winter air, the spring breezes, the moistness in summer showers, and the crispness of fall afternoons.

Thank you *heart* for your hard work through all of life's adventures—pumping ceaselessly, loving and sustaining me every second of every day.

Thank you *stomach* for transforming the food I ingest into needed energy.

Thank you *womb* for blessing me with a beautiful daughter and making me a mother.

Thank you *breasts* for nourishing my daughter through her first year of life.

Thank you *arms* for allowing me to hold close those I love.

Thank you *fingers* for allowing me to create, experience, and caress.

Thank you *legs and feet* for carrying me to the tops of beautiful mountains.

Thank you *body* for your diligence, loyalty, and love. You allow me to live and love completely. I am blessed to have you and look forward to our lifetime together.

# An Inner-Beauty Regimen

## Susan Law Corpany

Many years ago I was looking forward to a landmark high school reunion. With plenty of time to accomplish my goals, I started my pre-reunion diet. I tracked my progress not only on the scale but by tracking my measurements. When I proudly announced to my teenage son that I had lost a quarter-inch off my ankles—that's a quarter-inch per ankle, mind you—he put his hand on my shoulder and said, "Mom, remember that this is the part they put in the ground when you die."

That started me wondering why, so many years after high school, we are still so intent on impressing those people. Is it because we associated with them during the turbulent teenage years when we all wanted so much to belong and be admired? What

**Susan Law Corpany** *attended Utah State University, the University of Utah, and is currently studying at the University of Hawaii at Hilo. She also claims to have an honorary degree from the School of Hard Knocks. She won first place in the Imitation Erma Bombeck Contest for her humorous story "The Ghost of Housework Past," and was a runner-up the following year for her story "Fictional Dirt." Both stories celebrated women who hate housework. Corpany has published four novels and continues to write on the big island of Hawaii with her husband, Thom. She has a son, a stepdaughter, four stepsons, and a beautiful baby granddaughter.*

does it say about us if we are still stuck in thinking that we are defined largely by how we look and how we are perceived by our peers?

Now that I've passed the half-century mark—okay, okay, so I've hit the speed limit—I've finally realized that I am not going to morph back into a twenty-five-year-old anywhere but in my imagination. (And possibly in my husband's as well.) I recently ran across a photo of myself at twenty-two on my first visit to these beautiful islands of Hawaii I now call home. I showed it to my five-year-old granddaughter. She said, "Grandma, you could get that skinny again if you exercised every day all day long." Personally, I'm not sure even that would do anything but blow a kneecap or pop a shoulder. Sure, I do my best to hold the line, but I've decided it is time to work on my inner beauty.

Here are a few things to ask yourself before your next high school reunion.

*Am I more charitable now than I was in high school?*
*Am I a good listener? Do I care about who these people have*
    *become or do I just care about impressing them?*
*Am I genuinely able to be happy for their accomplishments*
    *and commiserate with them about their setbacks?*

If not, there is still time to start working out spiritually before the big event. First, let's worry about fine lines. We should worry about the fine line between being kind and unkind, the fine line between right and wrong, the fine line between responsibility and irresponsibility. We should worry about lines we draw that shut people out. We should worry about lines we use when we are being less than sincere.

Rather than worry about being lighter, we should worry about having more light. An official of the Israeli government saw that light shining. While acknowledging that the administrators at the Brigham Young University Jerusalem Center were appropriately ensuring that Latter-day Saint students were not proselyting in his country, he protested, "But what are you going to do about the light that is in their eyes?"[1]

One year, I pulled out an old junior high school yearbook, and as I glanced through it, I was struck by the fact that I could see which students had light in their eyes. It didn't matter if they had funky hairdos or squirrelly glasses or if they were the good-looking kids. Try it sometime. There is just something in the eyes.

Forget using face cream to minimize your pores. We should be worried about minimizing the number of poor among us.

We should worry more about sagging spirits and less about sagging body parts.

We should worry less about having crooked teeth and more about having crooked habits.

We should worry about whether it is our patience that is wearing thin, not our hair.

We should not worry about love handles. Love handles just about any situation you can find yourself in.

We should be more concerned about our double standards than our double chins.

Did you know that you can give yourself a face lift merely by smiling?

If you start now working on your inner beauty, all day every day, you'll be prepared for the one reunion that really matters.

---

NOTE

1. In James E. Faust, "The Light in Their Eyes," *Ensign*, November 2005, 20.

## Beauty for Ashes

### Michelle Linford

My best friend was telling me she was sure I had an eating disorder. She and my other freshman roommates had been watching me all year, secretly reading nursing-program texts together and analyzing my symptoms. I'm sure I couldn't hide the shock I felt. Or the anger.

I protested. Didn't she see that I ate three meals a day? I never skipped meals. I never made myself throw up. I was not by any means too thin. I exercised. I was healthy. Fit. In control. Listening to her, I felt betrayed. They just didn't understand.

The truth is, *I* didn't understand.

I came to college bringing a tenuous relationship with my body. As a late bloomer, I was still smarting from the changes of puberty. For many years, I had been the girl who was skinny as a rail who could also eat like a horse (and I did). Being a mousy, thin, flat-chested kid didn't do much for my sense of womanly

---

**Michelle Linford** *lives in Utah with her brilliant husband and three amazing children. Nothing recharges her like spending time with her family, but she also enjoys volunteer work. She's the managing editor of* Mormon Women *(mormonwoman.org) and has been involved with various advisory committees through the years. Her "to do soon" list includes rekindling her love of choral singing.*

worth, but I *really* didn't know what to do with the rounder, softer body that emerged as my figure and metabolism changed.

One of my most vivid teenage memories is of me standing in a Kmart dressing room in distress. All I could do was cry as I stared at the reflection in the mirror. I hated my body. I hated that my mom couldn't just buy me slim girls' clothes and training bras anymore. I hated the fact that she and my sisters were all skinnier than I was. I hated feeling ugly and fat. Thin was a badge of honor in my mind, and I no longer wore it.

Imagine my elation when, through no deliberate action on my part, the simple busyness of the first months of college life found me almost ten pounds lighter. The attention my mom received years before when she had lost weight was now being showered on me. It was a heady time. I was once again part of the skinny club, but this time I was no pipsqueak. I was a woman. I felt beautiful. Noticed. Confident.

From that point on, the scale became my best friend. I started exercising regularly. I was meticulous about what I ate.

Except when I binged.

I would binge and then skimp on my next meal. And exercise. Hard.

After a binging episode, I would feel unworthy to take the sacrament. How could someone so unable to consistently manage her bodily appetites be acceptable in God's eyes? Once again, I hated myself, but now it wasn't because I felt fat. It was because I was obsessed with a fear of being fat and a certainty that a girl who could not control her appetite wasn't worthy of God's blessing.

That fear almost kept me from serving a mission. I watched a friend serve in a foreign country and she came home more filled out than I ever wanted to be. I remember thinking, "I couldn't handle that happening to me." But then I realized that "I don't want to get fat" was a poor reason to give the Lord for not serving a mission. Serving a mission actually planted seeds of healing for me as I grew closer to the Lord and felt His love for me.

Fear also loomed large as I thought of having children. Not only was I worried about my family history of big hips and weight gain, but I also distinctly remember the thought I had while visiting a good friend who'd just had her first baby: *How will I ever be able to be home with children all day and be around* all that food?

It was only years later I realized my relationship with food and with my body had completely changed. I had been given sweet release from the clutches of my eating disorder. To me, it was a miracle.

I know that heartrending problems aren't always removed, even if we strive for that exact blessing. But I cannot deny God's hand. He delivered me.

Sometimes the beauty is in holding on and fighting when you have no idea how to win the battle. Sometimes the beauty is in continuing to believe when you can't imagine things ever getting better. And sometimes the beauty is in doing our part and then waiting on the Lord. At some point, God picks up the ashes and gives beauty instead.

# Recapturing Beauty

### Jayne Preciado

We live in a world of physical senses. For me, sight is the strongest. I spent the first eighteen years of my life absorbing the standards of beauty set by articles, movies, commercials, billboards, books, television shows, magazines, and other media. Daily, I took in media assaults that dictated what I should look like. Without recognizing why, I began feeling worthless. I started believing I was beautiful only if I was more beautiful than someone else. I didn't know I was struggling against the beauty in myself.

I wasn't alone. It was rare that my friends weren't worrying about their appearances too. Just out of bed in the morning, we'd start complaining at the mirror. Then we'd be agonizing over how we looked in this outfit or that. Every few minutes we'd be adjusting our clothes. *Does this cover that? Is this sticking out? Maybe I should have worn something else.* And then on the way to campus, every person we passed would seem a source of judgment

---

**Jayne Preciado**, *a junior at Brigham Young University, is a musician, linguist, and closet feminist when she's not busy reading textbooks and saving the world one essay at a time. Born in Los Angeles, she is a true NorCal girl at heart who loves spending time with her family in Sacramento.*

about how we presented ourselves—especially on the stairs by the Richards (PE) Building. Especially if it was a guy we were passing. (How is it that we just *know* a guy is *wow!* when we haven't even seen his face?)

As the day lengthened, so did our lists: My thighs look so huge in these jeans! If I fluff my hair, how long will it stay before it's flat again? Why do I look like I just stepped out of a sweatshop?! Is that reflection really me? Why is this me?! The girls I wanted most to look like were gushing that beauty was so much more than looks. They could. Malibu Barbie would wag her finger and say the same thing to Tour Guide Barbie, I know she would.

I wondered about women in history. Did they feel the world was staring at them too, finding fault with their appearances? Given the political and economic status of women throughout time, I despaired. Were we destined to wage eternal struggles to be successful eye candy?

I'm half-Mexican, living in a primarily Caucasian culture. Being centered in my identity here hasn't come easily, especially when the word *Mexican* used in my presence often refers to something inferior. I am 5'6" and 180 pounds. I have fat fingers, a shapeless butt, and a scar on my eyelid that leaves a gap in my eyelash line.

Over the course of nineteen years I've learned that true beauty embraces all of me. I've had to expand my senses to see it. I've got beautiful eyes. I am an expert at applying makeup. I'm a talented musician. I laugh easily. I'm kind to others. I'm a capable, intelligent woman. I'm surrounded by people who love me unconditionally. I know who I am—for the most part.

Beauty cannot be captured even by perfect hair or a darling outfit. It sometimes comes to you disguised in social rejection or as an intimidating opportunity. Though we lose our ability to see beauty sometimes, beauty will win out. The strength in beauty refuses to allow us to be formed by cookie cutters. Cookie cutters are for children. Let us be women! Women with vision. Women who revel in what others might call imperfection. Women who recognize ourselves as capable of moving the world.

I am beautiful because I choose to believe it and that decision has set me free.

## *Mirror Images*

### Diane L. Spangler

When you look in the mirror, what do you see? Feel? Think? In my work as a psychologist and professor, many students I know express deep disappointment, anxiety, or anger about their bodies. Many are seeking to achieve a body that is different from the one they have. This pursuit of a different body can occupy a significant amount of time and energy. Some have a clear idea about what mirror image they are seeking; that is, who they would like to look like—typically a Hollywood celebrity. What underlies this desire for body transformation, however, is often a mirror image of a different quest. The quest is idiosyncratic—perhaps a search for a sense of worth, of meaning, or of connection, or a hope of acceptance, of progression, or of peace. However, in seeking after the image of another, one seldom gains what was

**Diane L. Spangler**, *PhD, is an associate professor of psychology at Brigham Young University whose research interests include depression, cognitive theory, cognitive behavioral therapy, and eating disorders. She was the 2003 recipient of BYU's Young Scholar Award and has published numerous articles and books, including coauthoring "Body of Faith: Religious Influence on Body Image and Eating Disorders," in* The Hidden Faces of Eating Disorders and Body Image *(Reston, VA: American Alliance for Health, Physical Education, Recreation and Dance, 2009).*

sought after but instead experiences identity theft. Stolen are time, energy, and focus that could be spent in more life-promoting, authentic ways; but perhaps more importantly, one is robbed of the self-awareness, knowledge, growth, and joy that comes from pursuing a body and a life that are uniquely one's own. We were all made different from each other for a purpose, a wise purpose. In explaining the diversity of gifts and of persons, Paul told the Corinthians:

"If the ear shall say, Because I am not the eye, I am not of the body; is it therefore not of the body? If the whole body were an eye, where were the hearing? If the whole body were hearing, where were the smelling? But now hath God set the members every one of them in the body, as it hath pleased him . . . And the eye cannot say unto the hand, I have no need of thee: nor again the head to the feet, I have no need of you. Nay, much more those members of the body, which seem to be more feeble, are necessary" (1 Corinthians 12:16–18, 21–22).

When I reflect on these scriptures, I am reminded that we each bring something different yet vital to the whole. We can only come to fully know of our vital uniqueness and of who we truly are through seeking the image and path of Christ and coming to understand the paradox of losing oneself for His sake in order to find oneself (see Matthew 10:39). The way to satisfy any of the yearnings of worth, identity, connection, progression, or peace is to seek Christ and be remade in His image. This remaking is not in the outward sense of the world but in an inward sense of spiritual development. Those whom I have met on this path do have an image but it is not the image for which the world clamors. It is an image of charity, peace, and authenticity. These are they who "have . . . received His image in [their] countenances" (Alma 5:14). Their presence is felt more than it is seen. They are people of purpose, of kindness, of character, and of genuineness.

Their images in the mirror are diverse but their countenances are similarly Christlike. Interestingly, mirrors not only encourage a deceptive self-focus but the very images they produce are themselves deceptive. The image you see in the mirror is actually a distorted representation of what you actually look like and who you are. Your mirror image is only one-half your actual size, and may be, as warned by Isaiah, an "image that is profitable for nothing" (Isaiah 44:10). The halving effect of mirrors may well be instructive in terms of representing only half of your being—in representing metaphorically only the temporal but not the spiritual. Mirrors cannot tell us much about ourselves.

These days, when I do look into the mirror, I hope to more fully see who I am, to more fully see the mirror image of Christ, and to be able to more fully see as we are seen and know as we are known (see 1 Corinthians 13:12).

# I Didn't Care

## Liz West

Throughout middle school, junior high, and high school, I didn't care what people thought of me because I didn't care about myself. Although I had always heard that I was a child of God, I found it hard to believe.

What I began to notice is that the most beautiful people I met were the most gracious. And I wanted to be like that.

I wanted to choose. To choose what I would do and what I would say and to become who I wanted to be.

I get out of bed now not because I have to, but because I want to live in today.

I want to talk to people in my new class or ward or workplace because I know that each one is remarkable.

For me, self-confidence and the feeling of being beautiful came when I knew what I wanted to become and started choosing it.

---

**Liz West** *is currently living in her native England. She recently graduated from Brigham Young University with a bachelor's in humanities and hopes to earn a master's degree in social work.*

# Redefining Beauty, Regenerating Beauty

## Kayla

Wearing the most lightweight shirt I owned, I was still sweating more water than could possibly be in my body. And yet, as I stood on that busy Vietnamese street in 100 percent humidity at 100 degrees Fahrenheit, dozens of women were passing me on foot and on mopeds wearing long-sleeve shirts and coats. Why? In Vietnam, light skin is considered beautiful and the women around me were desperate to protect their skin from the sun. Not me. I was suffering in a T-shirt. Yet in my own culture, I am chagrined to admit I am often a slave to other illogical standards of beauty.

In America, we pay to expose ourselves to radiation seven times more damaging than the sun for the joy of sporting a tan. Never mind that we are increasing our chances of getting skin cancer. It is beautiful by American standards, so it must be worth it, right?

When will this beauty madness stop?

When enough of us redefine beauty.

I suspect that beauty is actually created by love. I know that sounds trite, but hear me out. If it is true, we could have a beautiful world simply by making a more loving world. That seems worth at least looking at.

Here is my experience. There is something in loving people that is more powerful to me than the illogical physical beauty that culture dictates. Love radiates out and transforms both men and women into people whose beauty is unmistakable and alluring. I have seen love actually change how a person's features affect me. I perceive them differently—with more beauty—when I feel their love!

Lloyd Newell says, "Be generous with your love, and you will never run out of it. Love regencrates itself—it grows by giving." I believe beauty is the same way. Beauty regenerates itself—it grows by being generous with your love.

# Beauty with Each Passing Day

## Megan Armknecht

I am a giant fighter.

You might be thinking that this is a fairy tale and I have to scrub floors for my stepsisters and wait to be rescued by a prince. No, no, no. There are no deep blue eyes, blonde hair, or dainty ankles here.

Actually, the giants I fight look an awful lot like some of those fairy-tale princesses . . .

I don't remember when I first became acquainted with the giants, but by high school, they were everywhere: on television, on billboards, in magazines, even in the school hallways. Some of them were hiding among my friends. The giants offered me lies. They encouraged me to compare myself to other people and told me that I wasn't quite good enough. And even though I professed that I did not agree with their type of "perfection," a little bit of me believed it—enough to take the poisoned apples they offered me. And by eating those lies of inadequacy and worthlessness, I locked myself in my own tower of misery.

---

**Megan Armknecht** *was born in Utah and has lived in St. Louis, MO; Washington, DC; and Las Vegas, NV—finally returning to Utah. She is a Wheatley Scholar currently serving an LDS mission in Donetsk, Ukraine.*

I thought things would change once I got to Brigham Young University. I thought college would immediately give me wings to soar out of the tower. But as the first semester wore on, I became more and more miserable, and I finally locked the tower door.

When I came home for Christmas break, my mom noticed the misery showing in my face. When I explained that part of the reason was that I thought I wasn't beautiful, she didn't say anything. She did, however, make me go on a drive with my dad.

I was mad about it. It was awkward. I was determined not to talk.

"Mom told me that you don't feel beautiful," my dad began. "And I'm not going to try to tell you over and over again that you're beautiful, because I'm guessing that you still won't believe me. But I need to say it at the start: You are beautiful. And, you should also know, that if there's another word that I would use to describe you, it is *elegant*."

My head shot up at the word. To be elegant was even better than simply being beautiful. Elegance not only meant beauty, it meant confidence. I certainly did not feel confident, and I felt the weight and responsibility of the word my dad had used to describe me; a word I felt I did not deserve.

That night, I reevaluated my hopes and desires . . . and my confidence. I wanted that confidence, and that night I wanted it even more than beauty.

I thought back to the fairy tales I loved to read and remembered an obscure tale, *The Three Little Men in the Woods*,[1] in which a girl—because she was good and selfless—was blessed to become "more beautiful with each passing day."

I wondered how that could be. If you were to become more beautiful with each passing day, soon your beauty would be overwhelming. But the tales said nothing of overwhelming beauty.

*Beautiful. Elegant. Confident.* The words rang in my head and

I gasped, realizing something. The girl in the fairy tale became more and more beautiful simply because she became more and more confident with who she was! I looked in the mirror. I *was* beautiful. But I wasn't confident, and it showed on my face. I fell on my knees and prayed for forgiveness, to be forgiven of the self-pity that had brought misery to myself and those around me.

I cried for the years lost in self-pity, of waiting for vanity, of not trusting myself. I had forgotten that "the worth of souls is great in the sight of God" (D&C 18:10), and it pained me to realize I had forgotten who I was—a true heroine, a true princess of noble birth. Suddenly, I was determined not to let the giants win! I pleaded for God's help in defeating them.

It hasn't been easy; the giants' poisoned apples are everywhere. Sometimes I have to shake myself to wake from the enchantment. Every time I do, I'm finding out that I am stronger, more determined, and more graceful than I could have ever dreamed.

And, with God on my side, I am getting good at fighting giants.

---

NOTE

1. See Jacob and Wilhelm Grimm, *Grimm's Fairy Tales*, ed. Edna Henry Lee Turpin (New York: Maynar, Merrill, and Co., 1903), 99–107.

# Beauty in Zion

## Kristine Hansen

*Aged women are the most beautiful women I know*, I decided while serving in the temple. Their faces are wrinkled and their hair gray, but they radiate beauty. They may have crooked teeth and double chins, but their serenity and warm smiles welcome strangers. They show up to serve in spite of aches and pains, pure light twinkling from the clear eyes behind their glasses. If any of them had ever been vain about their appearance, perhaps they overcame vanity through years of service: changing diapers, doing mounds of laundry, cleaning house, caring for children day and night, and serving in Primary, Young Women, and Relief Society. Could it be that kind of beauty comes from a life of *consecration*?

Consecration is necessary to establish Zion, a community that has been established only a few times on this earth. Only consecration produces complete unselfishness. No one in Zion is poor—financially, physically, socially, emotionally, intellectually,

**Kristine Hansen** *is a Brigham Young University English professor who has six great sisters, one terrific mother, and two amazing grandmothers, none of whom were seduced by today's false and shallow beauty myths, yet every one of them is beautiful in her individual way.*

or spiritually—because the inhabitants of Zion have all things in common and seek each other's happiness.

Zion is not here yet. The world we live in now encourages us to compete to do better than others and to live for ourselves. In this world, "being beautiful" too often means becoming absorbed with appearance and spending time and money on being the "right" shape and having the right hair, the right clothes, the right jewelry.

But "thou shalt not be proud in thy heart" (Doctrine & Covenants 42:40), the Lord told the Saints of this dispensation. And, "If ye are not one ye are not mine" (Doctrine & Covenants 38:27). How can we have an eye single to the glory of God when one eye is fixed on the image in the mirror? How can we be *one* if we try to exceed others' beauty?

I recently learned that over three billion of the world's people live on one or two dollars per day.[1] The money we spend on cosmetics in the United States—eight billion dollars last year—would nearly pay for clean water and sanitation for those three billion people![2] And what happiness have our consuming values bought our children? A major retailer is targeting girls as young as eight with a line of cosmetics to help them stay young-looking![3]

Of course, we should all make an effort to be presentable, neat, and attractive. But when does our focus on attaining worldly beauty leave *wholesome* behind and create trouble for us? Elder Neal A. Maxwell observed, "Many individuals preoccupied by the cares of the world are not necessarily in *transgression*. But they certainly are in *diversion* and thus waste 'the days of [their] probation' (2 Ne. 9:27). . . . People too caught up in themselves will inevitably let other people down!"[4]

When we seek "first the kingdom of God, and his righteousness" (Matthew 6:33), one thing that will be added unto us is a spiritual beauty that will never fade but grow stronger with time. As we "let Zion in her beauty rise,"[5] our own beauty will rise with it. We will shine with the radiance that comes from unselfish lives just as temple workers do. And we will attract heaven to earth.

## NOTES

1. Available at http://www.2dollars.org/; accessed 14 August 2013.
2. Available at http://www.worldwatch.org/node/764; accessed 14 August 2013.
3. Available at http://theweek.com/article/index/211492/walmarts-anti-aging-makeup-for-8-year-old-girls; accessed 14 August 2013.
4. Neal A. Maxwell, "The Tugs and Pulls of the World," *Ensign*, November 2000, 36–37.
5. Edward Partridge, "Let Zion in Her Beauty Rise," *Hymns of The Church of Jesus Christ of Latter-day Saints* (Salt Lake City: The Church of Jesus Christ of Latter-day Saints, 1985), no. 41.

# Beauty in Simple Moments
## *Name Withheld*

When I was a teenager, my family moved frequently. Like many girls, I sometimes felt lonely and inadequate. It seemed I could never live up to the world's standards. However, in small moments with my family, I felt beautiful, even with my bushy hair and braces. My parents were like lots of parents, photographing big events such as birthdays and graduations. But in my memory the small events had the biggest impact: painting the house, taking a Sunday nap, walking the dog. In some way, these ordinary times helped me feel beauty.

One such ordinary time took place when I was about six years old on a car ride with my dad. We were giggling and asking each other silly questions. Then I asked him a serious one. "Daddy, do you love me?" He looked at me and said, "Sweetheart, I love you very much." From then on, I never wondered if he did. I still feel beautiful when I think of that day.

When we lived in Oklahoma, my older brother told me I should grow up to be like a particular girl he knew. She became my hero, and I felt beautiful when I followed her example. Five years later, she became my sister-in-law when my brother married her in the temple. Another time, I felt beautiful when my mom told everyone at our Young Women's New Beginnings program about my divine nature. She said she was proud of me and told me I was beautiful.

In Texas, my little brother cried when we watched *Saturday's Warrior*, telling me how grateful he was that he had been born in our family. I felt beautiful and important. When we lived in Seattle, another brother was learning how to drive an old car with a stick shift. My brother was grateful for the car and never complained. His attitude was beautiful, and when I was with him, I also felt beautiful.

Although my family's many moves sometimes made it hard to fit in with the changing social scene, as a family we drew closer. We experienced beauty in our interactions with each other and I learned that the beauty in relationships far outweighs any other kind.

# Recapturing Beauty: What Beauty Means to Me

## Emily Mangum

My BMI (Body Mass Index) says I am on the heavier side of healthy. My jeans are size 10. Some of the tags on my cardigans read "Large." I have come to believe that I am beautiful. And I am beautiful because I choose healthy ways of being.

My journey has not always been so happy or so healthy. In fact, I admitted to my husband just a few days ago that when I was in junior high I used to sneak into the pantry to eat chocolate bars, a few at a time. When my mom handed me a book about binge eating, I was scared. I wanted to disappear.

What does it mean to choose healthy ways of being? Working out for hours and never eating a potato chip? Popping vitamin C and looking great in skinny jeans? Not for me. Well, I do love drinking water like it's going out of style, and I do love salads for dinner. I am also turned off by fast food. I'm usually careful about portion sizes and snacking, but not always. I love Swedish fish. I wish we had a never-ending, giant-sized bag of Swedish fish in my house. I love to make cookies, and I often eat way too many. I love snack foods, and if I am in front of a TV it is likely

---

**Emily Mangum** *graduated from Brigham Young University with a bachelor's in public health. She currently lives in Boston with her husband and son.*

I will munch mindlessly. Sometimes I still say to myself, "I know I'm not hungry, but I really want to eat all the fruit snacks. They are so good."

So how am I choosing healthy ways? As a graduate in public health, I learned that "health is a state of complete physical, mental and social well-being."[1] So I look to all my ways of well-being. I start with daily spirituality. I nurture my relationships. I find time for the people and activities that mean the most to me. I relax and enjoy my time. I exercise regularly because I don't eat like a bird.

Your healthy ways may be different from mine, and your definition of beauty may be different too. But that's okay. I feel healthy and so I feel beautiful.

---

NOTE

1. Constitution of the World Health Organization; available at http://www.who.int/governance/eb/who_constitution_en.pdf; accessed 18 July 2013.

# More Beautiful Than He Thinks

## Name Withheld

Six months after our wedding, my husband and I gingerly approached a topic that was becoming obvious to both of us. He was not physically attracted to me. No, he was not gay. He was, however, embarrassed to be discussing with me feelings he didn't have for me. He felt shallow and ashamed. He was still certain I was the very best choice for a life companion, but he had never really thought of me as attractive.

There it was, hard evidence I was not beautiful.

I was angry and hurt. How could the one man I chose out of the whole world—the one who chose *me*—how could he tell me he was not attracted to me? Wasn't he supposed to cherish me? I couldn't stop thinking about it. In the mornings when I got out of bed, I felt especially unattractive. When I chose what to wear, I worried that the wrong outfit might make him turn away from me. I wondered if bad hair might generate feelings of frustration in my husband, who *wanted* to be attracted to me. I craved being beautiful to him, and I worried that this problem was somehow my fault.

Not surprisingly, my confidence tanked as I started to realize I might never be attractive enough for him, no matter how

84

hard I tried. My personality started hiding, sinking deep inside of me, out of range. We talked about divorce, but neither of us really wanted that. I think we both were hoping that some miracle would come along and make me attractive to him.

A miracle did happen. But it had nothing to do with what my husband thought about me.

During this time of deep pain and insecurity, I finally realized that I was looking in the mirror in my bedroom and the mirror in my husband's eyes instead of the mirror inside my heart. At some point, I remembered there was another mirror, and I took a long look at myself. Down deep inside me, a voice reassured me that I was actually beautiful enough. Strength I had forgotten welled up in me, and I knew that what my husband thought about my attractiveness was not all that important. I could value him without taking on his weaknesses, including his inability to see my beauty. Something changed in me that day. I wanted to keep that strength with me, and I knew I would have to choose to believe in my beauty, even if no one else did. I prayed to overcome self-defeating thoughts, to avoid hatred, anger, and jealousy, which always bring self-doubt. I quit blaming my husband for his blindness and began being good to myself. That is my miracle.

And although it doesn't change a thing, I just want to mention that last week, my husband began to cry. He apologized for how he felt about me at the beginning of our marriage. He says he has discovered that I really am beautiful. The problem was inside him. He can't believe he said those things to me. He says he thinks I am the most beautiful woman he knows.

And I already knew that.

# Feeling Beautiful

## Elisabeth Oppelt

As women, it is our right to feel beautiful.

And yet we resist it. If someone says to you, "You are really beautiful today!" what is your reaction? Do you allow yourself to feel beautiful? Or do you think, "Oh, you don't really know!" Do you find reasons to believe in your own beauty? Or do you find reasons to discount it?

I first thought about this in a theater class, when Eric Samuelsen, the legendary Brigham Young University theater professor, taught me something I would never forget: Most men, he said, believe they fit in the top 50 percent of the world's handsomest men. We snickered. Most women, he said, believe they fit in the bottom 50 percent of the world's most beautiful women. We sat still. Really? Most women believe they are less beautiful than half of the women in the world.

I looked around the room and noticed that every single

**Elisabeth Oppelt** *currently works for a library company, but her goal is to teach high school theater. Her passions include theater, feminism, potato chips, and earrings. When she isn't working, she writes for several blogs and one magazine, reads non-fiction and fantasy novels, works on theater projects, and provides communications support for a non-profit.*

woman in that class was beautiful. I thought about my sister, who struggles with anorexia and bulimia and who boggles my mind with her inability to see that she is beautiful (I've always thought she was the pretty one). I thought about a friend who'd recently returned from a mission. I'd been struck by how beautiful she was, and now I heard she was struggling with low self-esteem. I thought about my mom, who had spent weeks looking for a dress for my wedding and cried because she felt she looked terrible in everything. My beautiful mom!

All of these women deserved to feel beautiful and none did. I was no different. I was comparing myself to advertisements, to clothing sizes, to other women, to my ex-boyfriend's ideal, and not surprisingly, I kept coming up short.

As I sat in that class, I came to a decision. I didn't want to spend the rest of my life believing I deserved to fit in the bottom of anything so important as how I feel about myself! No woman deserves to feel she isn't beautiful.

I started looking at myself. I already loved my passion, my intelligence, my talents. And when I stopped comparing what I saw to something else and just appreciated myself, I found things even about my appearance that I liked, I mean, really liked. I began to appreciate myself. I started to believe there were things *about me* that were beautiful.

I can't begin to say how much that moment in Eric Samuelsen's class changed me. Sure, there are still times when I look in the mirror and think *I need to lose weight; Maybe I should change my hair;* or *I wish my skin looked smooth right there.* But now, instead of letting those thoughts sink in, I notice their negativity. Instead of letting them pass, I look back in the mirror and say to myself, *You are an active person! You have good hair!* or *Don't those glasses look great on you!* I may not be able to stop negative thoughts from coming into my mind, but I don't have to let them stay. I can do just what I'd do if a stranger told me negative things about my best friend. I can tell those thoughts that they shouldn't come 'round here, 'cause I'm gonna defend my friend. I like her. I like me. And I deserve to feel beautiful.

# Trying to See Myself

## Maili Black

I'm a looker. Or so I've been told. It's not uncommon for me to be approached, complimented, or whistled at. Twice in my life I have been told by men that I was the most gorgeous woman they'd ever seen. I really have stared into the mirror just to see what others have apparently seen. I can't see it.

Sometimes after staring a while, I'd decide that my eyebrows were rather nice, after all. And I really loved my hair. But my nose? My thighs? My butt? Who could look past those? I was convinced I was really weird and deformed and appealed only to people whose view of beauty was deformed in the same way.

I'll tell you why I never saw that beautiful girl. I am not tall, thin, and blonde.

I do not have perfect lips, hair, legs, skin, etc.

I thought beauty was perfection and perfection was beauty.

Here's the lowdown.

Half of my genes are Cuban. I don't look like white girls or Hispanic girls.

I have a tiny waist and a big butt. And I have big thighs to go

---

**Maili Black** *is a Cuban and a momma. She is also a true blue Washingtonian who is crazy about natural health and loves her Father in Heaven.*

with that big butt. I see myself now as unique. But I started out, as I said, feeling weird and deformed.

My hips started to widen when I was thirteen. I had a tall, thin, blonde cousin who expressed how sorry she felt about my big butt. I cried myself to sleep over that.

I laugh now, because I love my body, but that doesn't mean it was easy. What I know now is that I would love to look like I did then for the rest of my life! I am healthy and I love my body. What's more, I'm happy and I am a confident woman.

So what's the secret? Why can I accept the body that at one time was my curse? Honestly, it's because I discovered that beauty is about what is shining through a woman, not what her body looks like. I like looking for the shine in women now, including myself. It is beautiful.

# Vulnerability

## Name Withheld

When I was in seventh grade, a boy on my bus told me he thought I was ugly. It didn't make me upset. Unfortunately, I assumed it was a fact. So I did worse than getting angry and telling him to buzz off. I internalized his comment. Worse, I assumed unattractive people came with unappealing personalities and so started to doubt my own.

I'm not sure why I thought that looking beautiful was a requirement for being a good person. I'd love to blame movies, or fairy tales (the ugly beasts that turn out to be kind princes are generally guys—not girls), but something inside me decided I was unworthy as a person. Overcoming that assumption took the help of good friends and church leaders who reminded me that my personality—my whole person—was good.

As cheesy as this sounds, I felt better about myself when I fell in love. Filling up my soul with love for another person reminded me how good my soul actually is. Being invited to open my heart and personality to another person invited me to see myself as lovable in ways I hadn't done since the seventh grade. At times, I was truly petrified of being seen and known. I remember shaking in the shower, realizing how vulnerable my heart would now be to being broken. However, I found out that I could be loved for—not in spite of—the quirky things that make me who I am.

I am beautiful, and I don't feel vain in saying it. I am not pretentious, nor am I full of myself. I simply like myself. My willingness to love and be loved makes me beautiful.

# Beauty Is Being Real

## Missy Jenkins

The minute I saw my mother, I knew exactly what I had learned in my first year of college. My mother was the most beautiful woman in the world because she was the most real woman in the world. When I walked into my house for the first time in four months, the only thing I wanted to do was hug her. As I held her tight, she smelled of warm vanilla and brown sugar. She felt soft and welcoming.

Although my mom exercises a couple of times a week, she has never had a dominating priority to have a smokin' hot body. She doesn't aim for having the skinniest legs, most toned arms, or the flattest belly. She doesn't worry about competing with anyone else. Her body is natural and simple. And I love that. And I love that she is soft. That's how moms are supposed to be. My mom is natural. And simply beautiful.

My roommate prides herself on her enormous hips. She says

---

**Missy Jenkins** *is a junior at Brigham Young University studying history teaching. She was born and raised in Idaho, and yes, she has grown potatoes. As the youngest of six, she has a lively personality, incorporating a mix of fabulous stuff from her older siblings. Missy's stubborn belief in herself (both physical features and character traits) has helped her find happiness in the full splendor of womanhood and motivate others to find that path too.*

they were made for childbearing. Sometimes I catch her lying on her side, running her hand along her oh-so-nice hip, saying out loud, "Man, I just love this!" Society tells women that large hips are not ideal and that looking stick-thin is sexy and normal. But she has her own ideas. And I am convinced that though she looks like no movie star, she looks like a goddess. She is beautiful and real.

My grandma Donna is aging naturally. Grandma is poised, graceful, classy, and elegant. She is seventy-eight years old but acts like she's sixty. I love her silver hair, big, bright brown eyes, and rosy cheeks. She has never had a facelift, botox, liposuction, or any other artificial treatment like that. She has just . . . aged. Grandma has deep wrinkles, especially when she furrows her brow or smiles her beautiful smile. I love those wrinkles. They are natural, and I think she is simply beautiful.

I want to be like my mom, my roommate, and my grandma. I want to be simple and real. That is beautiful to me.

# My Beauty Is My Family

## Mikayla Fuge

I am not a mother. I am not a wife. That part of my life hasn't come yet. But here's what I know. When I go home, I play Monopoly with my little brother. I run and play with my eighteen-month-old niece, coaxing her until she says my name. My six-foot-tall fourteen-year-old brother bear hugs me and won't let me go until I'm laughing so hard I can't breathe, and after a few days my youngest brother starts to run away from me because I have hugged and kissed him so much that he is afraid of being smooched to death. Every time I come home, my seamstress mother makes me a new long skirt to wear in the Utah cold, and my little sisters teach me how to do a new craft. I know next time I come home, I will take a trip to my favorite restaurant with my parents, and my older sister will take me out for a photo shoot. These things make my life beautiful.

My father's pride in me is the reason I strive to do well in

---

**Mikayla Fuge** *is a children's literature enthusiast in search of the perfect library. She loves to bake cookies, cakes, and pies, and unfortunately eats more of them than is really healthy. She has a strange love of dinosaurs and would like to meet one someday. For now she will have to settle for coloring pictures of them.*

school. My mother's love motivates me to serve. My older brother's dedication to his wife and daughter makes me want to marry someone who honors his priesthood as he does. My sister's skill as a photographer inspires me to develop my own creativity. My younger brother's quiet strength reminds me to endure to the end. Our family jokester helps me remember my days are better spent laughing than worrying. My younger sister's fashion sense reminds me to take the time to make myself look nice, even on the busiest of mornings. My brother's enthusiasm nudges me to be more excited about life. My youngest sister's sweetness hints to me that I can always be a little more loving. My family does not just love me—they remind me what it takes to be *beautiful*.

# Strength Is Beauty

## Mallory Hutchings

I find beauty in overcoming hardships. When a woman struggles, but still shows kindness and hope, she is beautiful.

My little sister Whitney was diagnosed with leukemia at the age of two. I can still remember how I found out. The kids walked into the children's hospital and sat down in a brightly colored room with animals painted on the walls. After what seemed like ages, my dad walked into the room with a tired smile and the word *leukemia* fell out of his mouth. Tears rolled down my face as I pictured my sweet little redheaded sister with such a disease. Anger, sadness, frustration, and worry exploded inside me. Why couldn't any of us protect her from this?! My dad said that Whitney was anxious to see all of us, and invited us into her hospital room. We had to dry our eyes so our distress wouldn't alarm her. Her tiny little body looked lost in the huge bed, and her happy face looked out of place.

---

**Mallory Hutchings** *grew up in the Seattle, Washington area. She loves music, art, reading, and writing and participates in many athletic activities. She is pursuing a degree in history teaching and art education at Brigham Young University. She is currently serving a mission for The Church of Jesus Christ of Latter-day Saints in the Canada Toronto Mission.*

My life spun out of my hands from that moment. Chemo-therapy treatments began immediately, and my dad had to be working every day, so it became my job to take charge of the house and the kids. Friends didn't figure in my life anymore and even school was far from my mind. The only thing that mattered was all of us making it through this alive. I was certain Satan had brought this upon my family, and it helped to be able to hate the cause of Whitney's sickness. Over that summer, she nearly tripled her weight thanks to steroids and lost all her red curls. When that precious smile of hers appeared now and again, I was buoyed up and would try to believe that she would live through this. Doctors told us that the cure rate for her leukemia was high, but getting there wouldn't be easy. Whitney endured more infections than I could count. She suffered seizures, kidney stones, hair loss, weight gain, immobility, loss of muscle mass, innumerable drugs and toxins, and more pain than I could imagine. She was the strongest person I'd ever met, and she was only two years old.

Just when the doctors started using the word *remission*, I was diagnosed with clinical depression. I hated doing everything. I hated going to school and coming home. I hated going to sleep at night because I knew I'd have to wake up to face another day. I remember wondering if anyone believed in me. And I remember deciding to believe in myself. I'm still not exactly sure how that happened. But I don't suffer from depression anymore.

My sister Whitney is the most beautiful person I've ever known, and some of that beauty comes from the strength she developed during her battle with leukemia. My depression re-minded me that, like Whitney, imperfections bring out strengths. When we accept our imperfections without resenting them, we are beautiful. When we reach for hope even when all seems hope-less, we are beautiful. When we are kind to others in spite of our pain, we are beautiful.

# His Pearl

## Name Withheld

Fireflies appeared in the twilight as we waited for the testimony meeting to start at girls camp in Tennessee. Always too shy to stand up at testimony meeting on Fast Sunday, I had promised myself I would stand up tonight. In my oversized, bright-colored T-shirt and with frizzy, unwashed hair, I stood and started to speak. To my surprise, I found myself witnessing the reality of the Atonement of Jesus Christ.

Walking back to my cabin afterwards, I couldn't stop crying. My heart felt as if it had been lit aflame with the love of God. Never had I known it was possible to feel such love. In that moment, there was no doubt: I was a royal daughter of my Heavenly Father. Jesus Christ had personally atoned for my sins, and God loved me beyond the extremities of my comprehension. When I think of Beauty, I think of that feeling, that sureness, that belonging, that divine nature.

Throughout the years, I have thought upon those spiritual highlights of my Tennessee summers. The memories are so moving and profound that they have become pearls to me, pearls from a loving Father, collected and strung together on a necklace that I finger whenever I feel inadequate in measuring up to the standards of the world. My necklace of pearls reminds me that beauty is available to me here and now from my loving Heavenly Father.

How do I reconnect with it? A girls camp quote about beauty helps me: "No amount of time in front of the mirror will make you as attractive as having the Holy Ghost with you."[1] This hit me as a teenager because I felt like I was always playing catch-up with other girls in the attractiveness department. Pictures reveal the perpetually bad haircut and the extra pounds which I thought were the main problem. But the real problem was that I hadn't opened my heart to the Lord's love for me!

Last week, I closed my driver's side door and braced myself for another long day on campus. I was struggling with a sense of being inadequate and stressed, and after too little sleep I was fighting to feel anything good. I wondered how I might possibly experience the love of God this day. Then I looked up—and there were the mountains! I wanted to let them sink in, to be overcome with their beauty in the sunrise. Oddly enough, I had to fight the sense that I didn't deserve to experience such love and beauty. Then the thought entered into my head:

*You are a princess.*

It was a voice I recognized—the same voice that supported me as I bore testimony and felt His love—the Giver of the Pearls.

I made the choice to surrender to that voice and let the beauty of His love sink into me. And because I did—despite my imperfections—God helped me remember that I am His beloved daughter. As I went about my day afterwards, I felt strong enough to serve others in my path. I noticed tender mercies. My problems and the consequences of my actions were not taken away—but I was on the path of love and beauty.

M. Russell Ballard counseled us, "Remember, eternity is *now,* not a vague, distant future."[2]

When I treat my day like a drop of an eternal life, I love myself more. I see myself as a daughter of God, not limited by the world's labels. I am not a singer, runner, or guitar player. I am a daughter of God who happens to do these things, but these things do not make me more valuable to Him. I am worthy because I exist.

I am beautiful and loved. *I* am His pearl.

---

## NOTES

1. Sheri L. Dew, "It Is Not Good for Man or Woman to Be Alone," *Ensign*, November 2001, 13.
2. M. Russell Ballard, "Spiritual Development," *Ensign*, November 1978, 66.

# Beauty as Reality

## Rachel Rueckert

I am exceptionally normal. My hair is somewhere between brown and blonde, my eyes are nondescript, my skin sports some grown-up acne and trendy jeans are a pain for me to try on. Yet I am okay. Actually, I am beautiful because I am real.

When I was little I knew that. I would squeal with delight at the sight of my own reflection. Yet only a few years later, I found myself avoiding mirrors altogether. I believed there was something unforgivably unbeautiful about me. When I saw girls on billboards or magazines, I would silently confess, *That's not me. I am definitely not beautiful.*

Then something happened to me. I became a photographer. I still remember my first digital photography class and the fascination I felt about digitally altering the world. I could make everything more beautiful. I got skilled at whitening clients' teeth, removing scars, and increasing color saturation. And as I

---

**Rachel Rueckert** *identifies as a cheeseaholic and wanderer. She is most interested in lifelong learning and education reform. When she is not enrolled in classes, gallivanting around the world, or teaching school in Massachusetts, she enjoys rock climbing, surfing, photographing, oil painting, reading, writing, and having meaningful conversations.*

worked in the business, the demands for beauty-enhancing work increased. I started doing more wrinkle erasing, touching up skin tone anywhere in the photo, changing eye color, and slashing off whole sections of people's anatomy in a kind of digital liposuction.

The fact was, every time I met with a client and discussed digital alteration, I was guilty of collaborating in telling them they were unacceptable-looking. "You want to change this? I can do it. Yeah, that looks like a little bulge; I can take care of that." Nobody's face or body was good enough. Believing that lie every day started dragging me down. I started to hate my work. Editing photographs was making me nauseated.

It got so bad that I started to avoid finding new clients because I didn't want to end up in a conversation with them about what was wrong with how they looked. I finally figured out how to manage this editing dilemma and it has changed the way I work. I now tell clients up front that I will no longer alter skin texture to make people look like plastic Barbie dolls. I tell them I won't remove wrinkles because I find character in them. My new copyright release form now reads: "I do not offer digital liposuction, nor permit clients to further alter images. You are beautiful the way you are."

We are real. We are flawed. We are unparalleled.

I finally believe that.

# First Lady

## Sarah Patten

Oh, what an honor it would be to be included in "The Top 10 Most Glamorous People"! And of all the famous and glamorous people in the world, it would be most amazing to be First Lady of the United States!

Since the day my first-grade class planned to present a play about presidents and first ladies, I have been intrigued. I saw quickly how a woman's talents and personality were valuable as a first lady. My favorite one was Lucy Hayes. Though I never saw her picture, I was convinced of her beauty as soon as I read my line: "They called me Lemonade Lucy because I didn't allow alcoholic drinks in the White House." I wanted to be courageous and beautiful just like her.

Finally the night of our first-grade performance came. I was so proud of my long pink sleeves and the bows on my dress. Though I was self-conscious about my glasses, I forgot about them as I anticipated my turn at the microphone. I wanted people

*Sarah Patten is a writer and educator. She enjoys learning new things. Her recent project was a fashion line called Recycled Chic. Her favorite piece of the collection is a skirt constructed from neckties sewn together, which her wonderful family contributed. She lives in California with her dog.*

to see me, to hear me. I had something to say! I hoped it would go as I had rehearsed.

Suddenly, it was my turn. I strutted to the microphone, said my lines, and then danced off stage. I had done it! Perhaps I really was a first lady at heart. And it wasn't just the costume—it was the fact that I had said something with conviction, and the statement reflected my beliefs. I felt courageous and beautiful indeed!

It's been eighteen years since I was Lemonade Lucy, but I'm still finding ways to be courageous. And that's how I find beauty. Doing what's hard—being courageous—makes me the first lady in my very own life.

# When Your Words Are Beautiful

*Melissa K. Condie*

My friends called me "Beaver" for a day in third grade in honor of my big front teeth. It hurt, and I remembered the name long after everyone else forgot. Then came glasses, braces, and headgear. I often wondered if I would set off the airport metal detector. I was also timid and scrawny, the kid everyone aimed to run through when we played Red Rover. So I learned to accept my place: I was not the girl that the boys would have crushes on. I was not the girl who wore trendy clothes. My hair would never behave.

That is why it was such a surprise when someone came up to me at a youth activity and told me I was beautiful.

"What?" I exclaimed in disbelief.

She seemed surprised that I was surprised. "You are so pretty!" she said. "Not only are you smart, but you are beautiful. You have it all! I'm jealous."

---

**Melissa K. Condie**, *currently free of braces and occasionally glasses, just got her first orchestra teaching job in Houston, Texas, after a few months of job-offer drought. With this opportunity, she will kick her bachelors in music education and master's in instrumental conducting into full gear. She is definitely smiling as she moves toward her dream life.*

Jessica, like me, was thirteen years old. She had been baptized into The Church of Jesus Christ of Latter-day Saints a few weeks before. I could hardly believe she meant what she said, but I wanted to believe it.

What if she was right? What if what was wrong with me also somehow made me beautiful? What if, instead of being nerdy, I could be smart? What if, instead of being scrawny, I could be slender? It started me thinking that maybe my weak spots could bring out good things in me.

Some years later, I had plans to meet friends at a concert of local bands. Not one of my friends showed up. I was on my own. I felt awkward, almost as if I didn't belong unless I was with someone. I wondered if I should leave. Instead, I found a seat next to people I didn't know and decided to introduce myself. I started to relax and found it easier to talk with my new acquaintances in between songs and sets. After the concert, we were parting ways when one of my new friends said, "You have a gorgeous smile. It was the first thing I noticed about you tonight."

Even though I never saw my new friend again, I never forgot those words. They give me even more courage to reach out to new people in awkward situations. Those words were beautiful.

So who can you empower by lifting them up with your words? Whose smile can you comment on? Everyone has a gorgeous smile.

When your words are beautiful, you are too.

# The Journey Is Rough

## Charlotte Marie Neeley

Discovering my own beauty has been a difficult journey.

I was eight when I started feeling ugly. I asked my grandma for some Oreo cookies after school. Mom usually gave me four, but Grandma only gave me two. I protested. She said, "No, Marie, you eat too many snacks, and you're gaining too much weight." That was it. I never knew my appearance mattered like that. I felt ashamed. As I look back on it, I recognize that I was hitting puberty earlier than my peers. I'd love it if I could change Grandma's words to "It's about time for us to think about a training bra for you!" or "Let's plan a nutritious dinner together," or anything positive about my life. Instead, I carried the sting of her negative evaluation . . . and started expecting more negative comments from other people.

And they came. I hated them. If I could just stop gaining weight, I could get rid of them. I tried to throw up after meals,

---

**Charlotte Marie Neeley** *is the oldest of four children. She lived in eight different states growing up with an Army dad. She met her amazing husband on a blind date at Brigham Young University and now has two incredible daughters. She and her family live in Ohio, where she tries to teach her girls every day how beautiful they already are.*

because that would solve my weight gain problem, but I could never gag successfully. I would give away most of my lunch at school, then exercise after school for two hours. I threw myself into clubs and activities just so I wouldn't have time to eat. Then when I got home, I'd tell my parents I already ate. Some days I would feel so anxious and starved, I would eat everything in sight. Then my father would scold me, "If you keep eating like that you'll get so fat you won't be able to get out of bed in the morning; is that what you want?" What I heard him say was, "If you keep eating, you'll keep getting fat." And so I very much wished I could just stop eating altogether.

Among the first questions asked when a baby is born is, "How much did she weigh?" I have a baby of my own now, and I worry that the carefree happiness she feels now about her body will transform into critical dissatisfaction when she enters puberty earlier than her peers, as she will likely do. I hate to think of her growing up with negative thoughts about her beautiful body. It will start with a well-meaning family member or doctor who will remark on how big she's getting. Maybe they'll tell her she's putting on a little pudge. They'll shower her with advice: She needs to exercise more; she needs to eat less or eat healthier; she needs to diet. She needs to get out of the house and play so she stops gaining weight.

That's right. Read that again; I said, "Stops gaining weight."

Of all the goals an eight-year-old should have, trying to stop gaining weight is not one that will help her blossom.

It's taken me until now, seeing a counselor and starting my own family with an amazingly supportive husband, to understand what happened to me more than fifteen years ago. How damaging talking about weight and size and shape with our daughters and granddaughters can be! When girls' bodies change, they are still beautiful. How many lives could we have saved from eating disorders if we had told our daughters, sisters, girlfriends, and other women that they are beautiful while their bodies are changing?

I plan on telling my daughter every day how beautiful she is. Even when her body is growing in new ways. Even when she's frustrated that her pants don't fit right or she doesn't look like somebody else. She is beautiful. And I am, too.

❀

# The Beauty Is in Me

## Heather Gemperline

I wear my midnight blue dress once a year around Christmastime. Add glossy heels, textured stockings, flashy earrings, a French twist in my hair, and a dress coat and I am good to go. I feel lovely enjoying the compliments that always come, and this year I'm looking forward to them. I need help believing I am beautiful in any way.

My heels click as I walk and swish into this year's venue to parade my Christmas dress. But this time it is different. No one talks to me; no one compliments me. My sense of being glamorous and wonderful appears to have been made up in my mind. I have to ask myself: *Am I less beautiful because no one says so?*

I remember well how my small wind of confidence was swept away in a tornado of despair. I just wanted to be told I was beautiful. But I felt humbled as I returned home. I remembered a scripture from the gospel of Mark. "That which cometh out of

**Heather Gemperline** *is a dance education student at Brigham Young University from Farmington, Utah. During her time at BYU, she performed in Jamaica and conducted dance research in Ghana. Though she loves traveling, Heather also enjoys making a difference through dance at home. She serves on the Utah daCi (dance and the Child international) board, organizes days of dance for children, and works at the BYU ARTS Partnership.*

the man, that defileth the man" (Mark 7:20). I thought *Maybe it isn't my outward appearance that makes me beautiful, it's what I bring to the world through my actions. Can I create beauty now in some other way . . . even though I am struggling with my confidence?*

This was my next thought. *I can love everyone I walk past. I can share that love with a smile. I can give a smile instead of waiting for the world to admire me.*

The first woman smiled back at me and walked past. A few steps beyond, she turned and called out to me, "Love your dress!" I was instantly gratified and had to remind myself that sharing my love with a smile was not simply a new way to get compliments, but a new way of being in my world. A group of three girls approached next. I practiced my theory again and smiled right at them. "Gorgeous dress!" one said back to me.

Remembering the lack of connection I felt at the Christmas event, I was astounded at the responsiveness of the strangers I was passing. Could it be that my loving act of smiling was actually making me more beautiful? I looked ahead as I passed the next stranger. No conversation, no connection. I went back to feeling warmth and love and sharing it in my smile and found the world a marvelously friendly place. As I finished my walk three more people approached. I smiled at each one and got smiles back that lifted me. By the time I reached my doorstep I knew that, just as Mark says, what was coming out of me was creating a truly beautiful woman.

The amazing thing is that when I took off the dress, I knew I was still the same beautiful woman. I wasn't worried about losing what I'd gained. I can give it to the world whenever I wish. The beauty is in me.

# Being Beautiful

## Kayla Merriman

What *is* beauty?

"Beauty is the gift from God."—Aristotle

My journey to discovering my personal beauty began when I was about eight years old, an age where every girl wants to (and perhaps should) feel like a princess. Girls often dream of fairy-tale lives, ending with a happily-ever-after and a handsome prince. When I was eight, however, I never felt like a princess. I didn't feel I had a right to imagine being one. I wasn't pretty enough and I knew it.

Growing up in the LDS Church, I learned about being a child of God and having individual worth. I was taught that every girl, as a daughter of God, is a princess and is beautiful in His eyes. I knew *about* these principles, but somehow I believed they applied to everyone else but me. These feelings started when my mother decided she wanted new experiences that did

**Kayla Merriman** *is a full-time mom finishing her bachelor's degree in communication disorders. She and her husband share a love of their daughter, missionary work, genealogy, music, and dancing. Kayla believes that life experiences are to be shared so we can help others. She lives by the truth that a little bit of faith goes a long way.*

not include her six children. She left when I was three, and I struggled with feeling worthwhile. After all, if my mom couldn't love me enough to stay with me, how could God love me? I often felt depressed. In high school, while on a European orchestra tour, alone in my hotel room, I wondered if anyone would notice if I just stepped off the window ledge.

Several years later, while cleaning out some boxes and papers in my bedroom, I came across a letter. It was from my mother, who still kept in touch, the year I turned eight. In it, she complimented me for good grades and expressed a desire for my brother and I to get along better. Next was her assurance that if I were to lose twenty pounds, I would be so much happier. I remember receiving similar letters and phone calls from my mother, each reminding me that I wasn't thin enough to be happy. Perhaps it's not surprising that I eventually developed an eating disorder which "helped" me drop a dangerous amount of weight when I was twenty and seriously threatened my health. Finding this letter so many years later reminded me of the pressure I felt to satisfy other people's expectations. Even when I reached the size I thought would allow me to be happy, I wasn't.

One afternoon, when I was twenty-one, I was stopped at a traffic light. It was a Sunday, and a morning of self-evaluation had left me desperate to feel something positive in my life. There at the intersection, I prayed. Somehow, I was—at this unlikely moment—ready for God to tell me who I was. Did He know me? Did He love me? I had to know. I hadn't prayed for anything in my life quite as intently as I prayed at that moment.

The answer came quickly, quietly, and powerfully. Yes, He knew me. Yes, I was His. Yes, He loved me and always would. Words cannot describe the feelings that flowed through me. I had never imagined being as beautiful as I felt in the car that day. God's love filled me with a beauty I had never imagined existed.

Suddenly I saw a future for myself that involved something more. God had a plan for me to do something *with* my life instead of just focusing on what was wrong with it.

Aristotle said that beauty is *the* gift from God. As we seek God and come to know Him, beautiful becomes *who* we are, not *what* we are. We recognize in us what God already sees—Beauty.

# Voice of Truth

*Brittany Butterfield Scott*

I've never felt pretty enough. I've always been a little too chubby, too white, too plain . . . whatever deficiency plagued me at the time. There was always *something*. I wasn't enough, but maybe someday I would be.

Then one night, not too long ago, everything changed. I was brave enough to ask a dear friend whose opinion I valued deeply, "Do you think I'm pretty?"

I don't know why I asked . . . But what he said changed me. And I will never go back to who I was before.

He looked at me, hard. With the intensity of that look came his answer as equally powerful. "You're *beautiful* . . . You're *gorgeous.*"

For some reason, I felt almost chastened by his words. Doubting my value was obviously my worst flaw. *I'd been wrong this whole time!* I'll never forget that night—that night when I for the first time considered the idea that my internal voice was

**Brittany Butterfield Scott** *is newly married and happy to start a new life with her husband, Geoffrey. She's passionate about music, theater, and food— but mostly people. If she were a Harry Potter character, she'd hope to be Luna Lovegood because every woman deserves to be that comfortable with herself.*

wrong. I could—and should—believe in my beauty, inside and out, and quit asking people what they thought about it.

Now it's my turn to tell you. You are beautiful. If you are listening to the voices telling you about your flaws and imperfections, if you feel that beauty is out of reach, I'm here to tell you the truth. It's high time you saw that questioning your beauty may be your worst flaw. Open your eyes, and tell everyone you know how beautiful they are.

Don't waste another day wondering what you're worth. You are beauty. You are love. You are life. Let that truth in now and let it transform you from worrying about yourself to sharing yourself.

You are beautiful. You always have been.

# Not Just Pretty

## Jennifer Ricks

The bright, Hawaiian-print skirt swished back and forth in the mirror. It was my own design, and even my thirteen-year-old brain could tell that it accentuated my short waist and awkward preteen figure.

"Mom, am I pretty?" I asked, still looking in the mirror.

She was behind me, marking the hem on my sister's similar dress, but she looked up sharply. "Yes!" she said firmly, almost fiercely with a couple pins clutched between her lips. "You are beautiful!"

This experience has stuck in my memory for a long time. As I look back, I think of what an awkward position I put my mom in with that question. For many years—during my teenage and young adult years of body image discovery—I thought she had lied. Of course she said yes, I would tell myself. She's my mom; she had to.

---

**Jennifer Ricks** *is a wife, mother, writer, designer, and musician. In addition to her pursuits, she enjoys engaging in all types of physical exercise, experimenting in the kitchen, challenging her husband to board game tournaments, and willing her thumb to turn green. You can learn more about Jennifer's writing and other creative projects at ByJenniferRicks.blogspot.com.*

But now when I think of this experience, I think more about myself, the questioner. "Mom, am I pretty?" I had asked. The question then was guileless, so different from the same question I asked years later of my roommate, and then my husband.

The truth is I'm not sure I ever asked that question aloud again. I was too afraid of hearing the wrong answer or not believing it if I heard the one I wanted. But I asked it of myself almost every day. I wanted to be pretty. I wanted to be beautiful.

I met my husband at a time when I would not have said I was my most beautiful. I was heavier than I had ever been, and the man I loved still fell in love with me. I got married without fitting into the small wedding dress I thought I needed to be happy. I survived a pregnancy and found that losing my normal body shape didn't take all the joy out of my life, like I once thought it would. I've adjusted to the long-term changes that motherhood has brought to my body and have embraced this as a new phase of beauty.

Since that day when I first asked that question, I have learned that *I am beautiful,* and it has nothing to do with the clothes that I wear, the numbers on the scale, my haircut, or my makeup style. The single thing that has made me satisfied with my beauty—no matter my phase of life—is being happy with my life.

Today when I look in the mirror, swaying side to side once again, I know I am beautiful. I am a reader. I am a writer. I am a culinary artist. I am a graphic designer. I am an interior decorator. I am a musician. I am an organizer. I am a financial planner. I am a caretaker. I am a nurturer. I am a runner. I am a dancer. I am a supporter. I am a listener. I am a comforter. I am a friend. I am a wife. I am a mother. I am a daughter of God. I am a woman of faith.

Mom told me the truth all along. I'm not just pretty; I am beautiful.

# Beauty and Combat Boots

## Bethany Owen

For me, beauty began with combat boots.

The first day I wore them, my feet felt big enough to crush cities. They were the only thing I could look at all day—in all their broken-laced scuffed-toe glory—and I was mildly curious as to why my ninth-grade classmates weren't paying attention to the massive shock waves that went rippling through the floor every time I moved my feet.

The purple heavy-toe Doc Martens had passed through a long chain of garage sales, friend-of-a-friend's boyfriends, and removed cousins before they were given to me by a neighbor who told me "you can pull these off way better than I can." I was clutching the boots like she might change her mind and take them back at the time, and I took her words very seriously.

"You think I can pull these off?"

"Yeah, for sure."

"Why? I'm not like . . . *cool*."

---

**Bethany Owen** *grew up in Minnesota, where she developed a tolerance for lake water and subzero temperatures. She likes hair dye, traveling, comics, and combat boots.*

"Neither are these, they just seem like your thing. I dunno. Do you want them or not?"

Of course I wanted them; they were *perfect*. They were beat up, heavy, hideous, a strange shade of violet—and only half a size too big for me. There was a promise on the bottom of the shoes that they could run through oil, fat, petrol, acid, and alkali. They were awesome, and they were completely wrong for high school.

I waited three days to wear them. I don't know what I was so worried about, since I was safely in the wallflower category at this point in my educational career, but maybe that's what I feared: being noticed, being looked at. I remember staring at them the morning that I finally took the boots to school and thinking very fiercely, *I don't care what people think about them. I like them. They can run through alkali.* With that, I changed into skinny jeans. I wanted the world to see them in full, framed by my bony knees and pigeon-toed stance.

I got a few comments. Nothing like the flood of shocked and awed exclamations I was expecting—nobody shunned me or dumped pig's blood over my head at a critical social point in front of my peers—but I got a few compliments and a few weird looks. What surprised me is that I liked my absurdly heavy shoes so much that what other people had to say about them didn't matter.

The feeling grew on me. I still had plenty of self-conscious days then, and I still have them now. Sometimes I wanted to shrink into my favorite superhero T-shirt and erase everything I'd said that day, or I'd feel so painfully awkward that I'd keep my contact with other people to an absolute minimum. But being unaffected by what other people thought, or said, or wore was such a good feeling that I threw myself after it. I wore my boots all the time, feeling daily inspiration from those two combat-ready purple beacons under my desk. I knew that I liked the shoes, I knew they were what I wanted, and I discovered that I could think that way about everything if I really wanted to. I felt so much better about myself once I realized that I was in charge. I felt confident. I felt intelligent. I felt beautiful.

For as long as they lasted, the boots helped me bring my inner beauty to life. And after a while, I didn't even need to wear them anymore to feel that kind of beautiful.

# Beautiful at Every Stage

## Dorothea Williams

My hair is brown. My eyes are neither blue nor green. My complexion has never been clear. I wish my body were a different shape. But I have always wanted to be beautiful.

I take out a photo album and look back at my life so far. Here I am at sixteen. My eyes and smile reflect the good girl I was and the love I had for life. But I didn't think my body was beautiful. I felt fat. I didn't know I was wrong. I didn't realize it then, but my body was changing and I was turning into a woman. I was beautiful.

I look at a wedding picture. My eyes are sparkling with love and happiness. My smile is radiant. But I was still worried about parts of my body. Would my husband accept me and my imperfections? I wasn't sure if I was attractive enough. Would my husband really want me? I am amazed I worried so much. I was truly beautiful.

---

**Dorothea Williams** *believes baking, sharing, and eating chocolate chip cookies can turn even a bad day into a great one. She is a musician and journal writer and is grateful for modern technology, which allows her to share her four children with their grandparents who live across various oceans. She resides with her husband and children in California.*

Here is a photo of me, pregnant with the first of our four children. My face is glowing. I look excited and hopeful about this unknown adventure I am about to embark on. Yet with an extra fifty pounds of pregnancy weight I did not feel beautiful despite the miracle I was participating in. Why couldn't I see then how beautiful I was?

My beauty in each of these photos is obvious to me now. Why was it so hard to see past those perceived flaws at the time? What has changed?

I realize that I am blessed to be married to a man who for the last twelve years has told me, almost daily, that I am beautiful. There are times I believe him, and times when I think, *Really? You think I'm beautiful right now?* With a loving smile he replies, "But it's true! You are!" When I am feeling big in those fifty-pounds-heavier pregnancies, he says he sees me as a queen, sacrificing to bring our children to the world. He tells me I am beautiful when I wake up in the morning with messy hair and baggy eyes, knowing that I have been working hard on taking care of our home and children. Those things make me beautiful to him.

Having children also helped change my perspective on beauty. When my baby looks up at me with complete trust and love, when my toddler comes running to my arms for comfort, I realize I am the most beautiful person in the world to my children. Whose opinion could matter more?

It was somewhere between my husband's loving and sincere words and my children's sweet glances that a change slowly grew inside me. I decided I didn't ever want to look back on today, years from now, and finally realize I was beautiful even then. I needed to recognize it now.

That's when I realized that I am beautiful at every stage because I am fulfilling the measure of my creation. My body is changing and aging. But knowing I am fulfilling my mission on earth using the divine gift of my body makes me appreciate what a truly beautiful creation I am.

My hair is brown, with warm specks of gold and red that you can see when the sun falls on it. My eyes are blue-green and deep like the sea. My face radiates calm confidence. My eyes shine with joy and gratitude for life and for the woman I have become. My body represents strength, sacrifice, courage to fulfill my divine destiny and give warmth to those I love. All these things make me beautiful.

I no longer have to look back at old photos to see my beauty. I see it in the mirror. But more importantly, I now gratefully feel it every day inside my soul.

# Whenever I Feel the Rain on My Face

## Julia Sorensen

Nobody celebrates rainy days. When they sing about them, they're sad songs. But I love the rain. Let me tell you my story and you will understand why.

• • •

I leaned heavily on the bathroom sink, my knuckles white from gripping. My reflection in the mirror was hazy from my tears. There was no reason to be so scared of what I would see tomorrow when the bandages came off, I reasoned. All of the other surgeries had gone well; why shouldn't this one?

Since my first visit to the hospital, when I was born perfectly healthy except for facial defects, I'd been back many times. Minor facial operations were a part of every single one of my seventeen years. This one, however, promised to be the final installment in rearranging my face, and tomorrow the bandages would

---

**Julia Sorensen** *is a science nut who loves experimenting with pancake recipes and practicing Morse code with a keychain flashlight. She works as an intern in a hospital laboratory and is excited to be helping patients. She and her husband enjoy taking long walks and incessantly quoting movies.*

come off. I squinted through my misty eyes to try—*try*—to see through the sterile wrappings. How would it all look tomorrow, unveiled?

I confess I was overcome with apprehension in thinking about the final outcome, and those tears escaped. Part of me felt silly. I was healthy and happy, and so blessed that my lopsided nose could be completely fixed thanks to modern medicine. But a girl can't bury her insecurities beneath logic, however hard she tries. And so I cried out my worries. Then I closed my eyes and said a silent prayer to my Father in Heaven, asking for a small measure of His grace to bless my face, that it could be beautiful after all.

• • •

When I was fourteen, I had a serious nasal surgery. I remember visitors coming to see me as I recovered. They looked at me from a respectful distance and said, "Oh, you look so good!"

I hated it when they said that.

I was floored when I finally looked in the mirror. Twin black eyes stared out from swollen sockets, and the rest of my face was puffed up pretty bad too. My nose was stuffed with bloody gauze and my sweaty hair was plastered to my head. *This* looked good? I was mortified.

Just when I aimed to go sit on the couch and feel sorry for myself, Dad insisted I go for a walk. As we made a few circuits around the backyard, I clung tightly to his arm. The afternoon Texas sun shone brightly, making the whole world glow with soft warmth. My self-pitying mood began to lift, and I was glad I had come. My dad encouraged me the whole way, commenting on the fresh air, the sunshine, and the beautiful day.

"And you," he said, looking fondly down at me, "you are beautiful too."

It was different when he said it. I don't know how; it was the same sentiment I had tired of hearing from all the visitors. It was different because I knew he meant it. Somehow he looked at me and truly saw beauty.

•   •   •

Three years later, I still remembered what my dad had said that night. And as I spoke to my Heavenly Father there in the bathroom, I knew that He would say something similar if I could be so lucky as to walk with Him. He had made my face, and however it would appear in the morning, in His eyes I would be beautiful.

The next day, I wasn't even nervous as we drove to the doctor's office, but I was excited. As the nurse braced her scissors to start snipping at the crash helmet of bandages wrapped around my head, I shut my eyes and waited.

•   •   •

It started to barely rain as we left the doctor's office. On the way home, we stopped at an outdoor park of beautiful fountains and got out to enjoy the day. My face, which had been covered for so long, felt extra sensitive to the gentle rain. I couldn't help but close my eyes and feel the drops against my skin. With every drop, I felt the love of my Heavenly Father, who had known me since before my birth, who had made my body and guided my life. I felt His blessings and His care with each drop that landed on my nose: *perfect, perfect, perfect.*

❁

# Redefining Beauty for Myself

## Kelli Dougal

I looked out over the group of bright-eyed girls staring back at me as they promised to focus on positive aspects of themselves instead of negative ones. I smiled at them as they promised always to think of themselves as beautiful. But as I smiled, I felt like a hypocrite. I was teaching these girls to stop picking out their flaws when they looked in a mirror, but that was exactly what I had done earlier that morning.

It was ironic, really, for a pageant queen to be telling girls that there were more important things than looks. But as a local titleholder in the Miss America system, that's what I had chosen for my service platform. My platform, "Redefining Beauty," acknowledged that many women's problems stem from a lack of self-acceptance of their body image. I knew about these problems because I'd experienced them myself. In fact, as I stood there smiling at all those girls, I remembered that just that morning

**Kelli Dougal** is a recent Brigham Young University graduate facing the daunting task of figuring out what to do with her life. Her goal is to find or invent a job that involves her favorite things: writing, eating, singing, dancing, and giving dating advice. She currently resides in Washington but hopes to end up on the East Coast again someday.

I had cried while looking in the mirror because I didn't think I looked good enough to make an appearance that day.

It's easy to blame body image problems on the media, but my lack of self-confidence wasn't just the media's doing. I was the one who decided to participate in pageants where physical appearance is the first reason to be praised or rejected. Even when the pageant was over and I didn't need to worry about strutting onstage in a swimsuit, I still got distressed anytime my body didn't look like a pageant winner.

I didn't even realize just how much of my self-worth I based on my appearance until one day I found myself sitting in front of the mirror crying. I had applied my makeup, taken it all off and applied it again, but no matter what brushes I used, I just couldn't cover all my imperfections.

As I sat there crying, I realized something: I was being completely unrealistic. I wasn't a failure if my skin wasn't perfect! I slowly began to comprehend that I had slipped into a terrible belief system. If I looked good, I was happy with myself. If I didn't, I was unhappy. I could live a beautiful life, create beautiful music, and care for others, but if my skin wasn't clear, I felt defeated and angry. If people seemed distracted instead of interested in me, I thought it was because I wasn't attractive enough.

As I stared at myself in the mirror that day, I realized that I had been hiding behind my appearance. I had put so much time and effort into "fixing" my face and my body that I had forgotten about the other things that were important to me—I had forgotten about the things that made me *me*.

I decided to start practicing what I preached to the girls in my community: I needed to redefine beauty for myself. I made lists of admirable traits I possessed that had nothing to do with my appearance. I read old journal entries to remind myself of things I loved doing. I made an effort to spend time with people who were uplifting and who made me feel good about myself no matter what I looked like. Some days, when I wanted to cry because I was disappointed in the face in the mirror, I literally had to sing to myself, "Girl, you're amazing . . . just the way you are."

I'm still on a journey to redefine my beauty. At the end of my year of service, I passed on my crown; I no longer teach girls about inner beauty. However, I'm still teaching myself on a daily basis. I've begun to understand that I am a truly amazing person whether or not my eyelashes are curled or my skin is smooth. And I've really started loving the person underneath.

❀

# According to the World, I Am Not Beautiful

## Sadie Klein

My round face is not gracefully sculpted. Baby fat lingers around my middle. My hair has a stubborn mind of its own. I do not turn heads, catch eyes, or receive slipped phone numbers after brief encounters. To make matters entirely worse, I have no fashion sense at all.

The girls who stroll the beach in perfectly fitting bikinis? Yes, I hear *they* are beautiful. Girls with long, sleek hair and doe eyes? The ones who pose for magazines and look like they haven't eaten in days? The celebrities and movie stars that spend hours becoming presentable? Not only are they beautiful, they tell me that I am not beautiful.

Growing up like this has been crushing to my self-esteem. It was obvious from the beginning that a girl who played with makeup was far preferable to a girl who curled up on the couch with her favorite book. People made it known very quickly what

**Sadie Klein** *spends too much time idolizing Batman and Captain America. When she's not being a comic book nerd, she reads and writes with the hope of being an author someday. She can't wait to graduate from Brigham Young University with an English degree and go out into the world, learning how to be her own kind of superhero.*

they preferred, and I did not fit the bill. For a time, I couldn't look into a mirror without scorning the person staring back at me.

One day, I decided to stop thinking about myself and think about the beauty in others instead. And that was the start of my journey. I can't tell how I learned to appreciate my own beauty until I explain how I began to appreciate others. Noticing others came first.

The boy across the way? His ears stick out a little bit. It is adorable.

The girl who lives a few apartments down? She is one of the smartest people I have ever met.

The girl who I sit with during class? Her laughter is infectious and her eyes come alive when she smiles.

One of my very best friends? Her wit cracks me up.

None of these traits are beautiful in the worldly sense. In fact, the people I mentioned will never be supermodels, but they are more beautiful to me than any celebrity.

When I found the beauty in them, I also found that I was judging myself harshly. After a conversation where I compared myself to another girl, my friend asked me why I was shooting myself down. And you know what? I didn't know why. If I don't look down on other people because they're not perfect, why do I berate myself for my own imperfections? If laughter, knowledge, and ears that stick out can be beautiful, I can be beautiful, too.

I can talk about books for hours and share which ones are my favorites. I can gush about the way the words weave together to create imagery that whisks the mind away to fantastic places.

I can sing at the top of my lungs, although my notes aren't perfect. I can dance around the kitchen in my socks, though I'll never win a televised dance competition. I can laugh helplessly until my sides ache.

I can create worlds and towering cities with the things I draw and the words I write. I can tell stupid jokes that make people smile even though they scoff a little. I can greet someone with excitement that makes her believe she is the highlight of my day.

I can build friendships that will last a lifetime. I can be kind, charitable, and optimistic. I will probably never be a supermodel.

I will probably never turn heads, catch eyes, or have phone numbers slipped to me.

I will probably never fit into society's definition of beauty.

But I am beautiful, too.

# Scared to Be Pretty

## *Name Withheld*

From behind the steam, I saw my face emerge. At sixteen, I resented the chubby face, the white skin, and the thick hair that showed up every day in the mirror. As quickly as possible, I dusted on minimal makeup and pushed up my glasses. My hair went up to a twisted bulge behind my head. Done. Somewhere inside myself, I knew I was hiding. I was six feet tall and overweight. Everything about me seemed wrong.

I hadn't always been like this. Once upon a time, I skipped down the stairs, dressed up and dreamed of being an elegant artist. But that girl was gone. Nothing about me fit that dream anymore.

Once when my hair was wet, I didn't knot it up. As it dried, I could feel it expand into a puffy pyramid. Then my dad saw me. "Wow, you look pretty," he said with his hand on my back. That hand. That hand that lied. The one that could not stay away from pornography. My back felt like it was on fire under that hand. I didn't let my hair dry free again.

People always said my mom and I looked alike. Didn't he think my mom was beautiful? Was she beautiful enough? What was he looking for in the pictures? *I did not want to be what my dad thought was beautiful.* If being beautiful meant attracting someone else's dad and ruining their family, I did not want it. I was scared to be pretty.

I did admire my beautiful friend who had curls cascading down her back. One day, she told me we had the same hair, and I was shocked. I did not know I had curly hair! She let my hair down (literally) and introduced me to mousse, hairspray, and scrunching. More importantly, I began learning it was okay for me to be my beautiful self. Scary, but okay.

When I was ready to serve a mission, I got a call to the fashion capital of the United States: New York City. Despite its focus on beauty, glamour, and first impressions, it was there (of all places) that I discovered my Father in Heaven.

I walked the NYC streets with as much confidence as any beautiful person there, because my confidence was rooted in my Heavenly Father and His message. He worked a miracle in me and nourished the delicate seed of self-acceptance. I began to understand that I could choose my own happiness. I could choose to love me: His masterpiece.

An old friend wrote faithfully while I was away. He knew me back when I was defined by the bun, the chubby cheeks, and the glasses. He called me the day after I came home and persuaded me to move to Provo (where he was living) five months earlier than I had planned. He found an apartment for me that just happened to be in his ward, in his family home evening group, *and* he signed me up for his dinner group—all before he had even seen me!

He didn't know I had lost fifty pounds on my mission, stood tall in my six-foot frame, let my curls out more often, and had the makings of confidence. Our mission letters started in friendship and ended in love, and he saw my beauty the whole time!

I felt beautiful when he opened my car door, when he taught

me how to ballroom dance, when we kissed during a night stroll, and when he listened and stroked my shoulder while I cried.

I felt gorgeous the day we were married, whenever we gut-laughed ourselves to tears, and when he brushed a strand of curly hair away from my face after the birth of our daughter.

I trust him. I see his eyes pinned to our family—to me. I see him look into the eyes of his daughter and declare her *beautiful*. He knows what that word means.

Now, when I wipe away the steam from the mirror, I am more accepting and kind to my Heavenly Father's daughter. I still struggle in letting my hair down, but I know Heavenly Father is my real father, and He sees real beauty in *me*.

❀

# Believing That You Are Beautiful
## Kellianne Houston Matthews

*Nothing makes a woman more beautiful than
the belief that she is beautiful.*
—Sophia Loren

In junior high, I performed with a ballroom dance team. My mother custom-made my costumes because the school's collection was too small for me. One of our coaches pulled me aside and told me not to pay attention to the criticisms of other girls who wanted me off the team because of my size. "One day, you're going to be a beauty just like your mother," he reassured me. Yep, I was the ugly duckling.

The irony was that when that beautiful day eventually came when I achieved the size and shape I'd worked hard for, I still didn't feel beautiful. It hadn't changed a thing!

When did I start feeling beautiful? When I had to undergo

---

**Kellianne Houston Matthews** *is a firm believer that there is beauty in all that life has to offer, be it her adventure with brain surgery or the simple routine of walking her dog each morning. Kellianne currently lives with her husband and dog in Utah, where she enjoys keeping busy with education, art, design, psychology, animal science, and ethology.*

brain surgery, and I realized what life meant to me. It no longer mattered what size I wore or how much I weighed. Life was a gift far more precious than numbers could tell.

As President Dieter F. Uchtdorf explains, "Like this young swan [the "ugly duckling" from Hans Christian Andersen's story], most of us have felt at one time or another that we don't quite fit in. Much of the confusion we experience in this life comes from simply not understanding who we are. Too many go about their lives thinking they are of little worth when, in reality, they are elegant and eternal creatures of infinite value with potential beyond imagination. . . .

"My dear young friends, this knowledge allows you to see your own reflection in the water. It assures you that you are not ordinary, rejected, or ugly. You are something divine—more beautiful and glorious than you can possibly imagine. This knowledge changes everything. It changes your present. It can change your future. And it can change the world."[1]

It has taken me twenty-two years, but I finally have discovered that I was always a beautiful swan. Even when all I saw in myself was an ugly duckling, it will never change the fact that I am beautiful—I *am BEAUTIFUL♥*!

---

## Note

1. Dieter F. Uchtdorf, "The Reflection in the Water," CES fireside, 1 November 2009, Brigham Young University; available at http://www.lds.org /ldsorg/v/index.jsp?locale=0&sourceId=81e3f5036e881210VgnVCM100 000176f620a_____&vgnextoid=43d031572e14e110VgnVCM1000003a9 4610aRCRD; accessed 18 July 2013.

❀

# Feeling Beautiful

## Kimberly Chamberlain

I was ashamed of being a girl before I was thirteen. I loved Super Soaker wars, secret agent missions, and sports. I shopped for boys' clothes, kept my hair in a bob with bangs, and refused to wear makeup. (When a friend suggested a makeover, I hid out till she was gone.) Showering regularly, brushing my hair, and wearing deodorant were not important to me either.

Crushes struck me as particularly gross. Guys had always been my friends. If they stayed that way, I was fine. Their weird interest in girls made me uncomfortable sometimes.

Then in eighth grade, I became a percussionist and started private drum lessons with a guy two years older than me. I was afraid I would start crushing on him and tried my hardest not to think of him in that way. It happened anyway.

The first time I ever cared what I looked like was when our Young Women leaders took pictures of us all and lined the hallway bulletin board with them. That was *me?* My hair was a mess,

**Kim Chamberlain**, *who jokingly calls herself a "corporate brat," has lived in six states, mostly in the Midwest. She is a junior at Brigham Young University, hoping to double major in media arts studies and Spanish to pursue either a career path in the film industry or for a federal organization such as the FBI.*

my glasses were smudged, my sweater/T-shirt combo looked way too big, and my braces did nothing for my cheesy smile. The idea that my drum teacher saw me like that was mortifying.

I was motivated, but the change was gradual. I got my braces off at the end of the year and started shopping for girls' clothes. I grew my hair longer and started wearing makeup. And I started noticing guys. I also noticed that if I really liked a guy, he was hard to talk to. If I thought of him more like a friend, he was easy to talk to.

Why? Eventually I figured it out: I would act timid around guys that I liked, but I wouldn't be afraid to be myself with my friends. My true beauty came through when I was comfortable being myself.

So I made a vow. No matter how awkward it feels at first, no matter how hard it is to imagine I belong, I refuse to hide my true self. I take the advice in Matthew 5:16 to let my light shine. And when I do, I feel beautiful.

# I Dreamed of Becoming Beautiful

### Eun Si Re Song

I have always been fascinated by beautiful women in the movies. I secretly hoped one day I would become one of them. When I was a little girl, I was delighted to hear grown-ups tell me that when I turned eighteen, I would be beautiful. So on my eighteenth birthday, I sprinted to the bathroom first thing. Somehow I was sure I would see something beautiful in the mirror. Such disappointment! It was just me.

One of the beautiful women I actually knew was my mother's sister. I didn't see her very often, but I had memories of her cooking delicious foods and smiling her beautiful smile at me. When I graduated from high school, my mother and I decided to celebrate by visiting my aunt in Korea. On this visit, I looked at her with new eyes and realized that in spite of my intense experience with her as a beautiful woman, she wouldn't necessarily fit the world's standard of beauty. I wondered what it was that

**Eun Si Re Song** *is pursuing her interest in international business by studying international relations at Brigham Young University. She is dedicated to learning about different types of people and wishes students the happiness of doing well in school.*

continued to captivate me about her. Why did she convey beauty to me, despite not matching the movie-star ideal I had come to value?

Then I learned my aunt's story. When she was born, she suffered some genetic defects that doctors elected not to correct. She developed an abnormally shaped body, amorphous facial features, and crooked teeth. Because of her appearance, she got used to people pointing at her and making rude comments. People she might otherwise have called friends made fun of her. She went to college and tried to ignore the fact that my mother and two other sisters had active social lives and seemed very popular. Gradually, the stress of looking different and being treated demeaningly took a toll on my aunt and she withdrew into her own world. My mother told me that for a long time my aunt rarely went outside.

Then one day, she took courage and went for a walk. At a nearby park she was moved by the homeless people she saw. Something inside her started to change, and she began to see how she could make a difference with her life. She started studying for the public servant examinations available in China and eventually secured a job at the welfare institute. After twenty years of public welfare service, she was in a position to establish a care center for homeless people. Shortly thereafter, she started a center to provide education to low income children. She is still the head of that center and still devotes her time and attention to people who have great needs.

Today my aunt is a very respected person in her community. She has earned the trust of the government and the people. When I see the work she does to feed the homeless and to teach underprivileged children math skills, she is extraordinarily beautiful to me. She shines.

❀

# Perfection

## Mary Caroline Richards

To be perfect
even as your Father in Heaven
is perfect . . .

How, O God, am I to understand
the word?
Perfect and pure in heart?
What means pure?
Pure, pure,
Pure apple juice!
I begin to sense a clue.
Pure apple juice is made
from the whole apple;
bruises, blemish, skin, core—

---

**Mary Caroline Richards** *(1916–1999) was an American poet, potter, and writer, best known for her book* Centering in Pottery, Poetry and the Person. *Educated at Reed College in Portland, Oregon, and at the University of California at Berkeley, she taught English at the Central Washington College of Education and at the University of Chicago. After serving on the faculty of Black Mountain College in North Carolina, she taught art at the Institute in Culture and Creation Spirituality at Holy Names College.*

the whole imperfect works.
Pure apple juice is not
pasteurized, refined,
filtered, nonentity!
Bruises, blemishes, skin and core.

To be perfect is to be
Whole, a paradox
Even as our Father in Heaven . . .

---

## NOTE

Mary Caroline Richards, "Perfection," from *The Crossing Point: Selected Talks and Writings* (Middletown, CT: Wesleyan University Press, 1973). © 1973 Mary Caroline Richards. Reprinted by permission of Wesleyan University Press.

# True Beauty

## Anna Finneran

There was a time when I believed beauty could be seen only with the eyes. That all changed when my mother told me a story. She was fifteen years old and got a job making fruit drinks. One day she saw a can of orange juice sitting in the hot frying oil, probably put there by someone who was attempting to defrost it in a hurry. As she fished it out with tongs, the can exploded, showering her with boiling hot oil. She was knocked to the ground, paralyzed by the force of the explosion. Her coworkers called 911 and the emergency team discovered her clothes had been melted to her body. When my mother arrived at the hospital, the doctors carefully peeled her clothes off, removing skin too. The doctor took my grandmother aside and warned her that my mother would never look the same again. Already her face had swollen to triple its usual size and her dark brown eyes had turned bright blue. She would stay in the hospital's burn center

---

**Anna Finneran** *is from California and Utah. She loves the outdoors and being with people. She loves to search out the "Why?" to every question and loves to sing. Currently she is serving a full-time mission in Paris, France. She will study French with a minor in Spanish at Brigham Young University when she returns. She loves the little surprises that life brings and most of all she loves her Father in Heaven and her Savior, Jesus Christ.*

four months, getting her skin peeled daily and enduring numerous skin grafts. Miraculously her face today shows no scar, which she attributes to the priesthood blessing she received during her first night in the hospital. The rest of her body bears multiple scars.

I had never considered whether my mother's skin was beautiful before I heard that story. I had, however, experienced her patience, compassion, and wisdom, which *felt* beautiful to me. So in the same moment I recognized the impact of her story—that her skin might not be called beautiful by the world's standards—I also recognized that my mother's patience, compassion, and wisdom had been deepened and refined by her ordeal. Her true beauty increased and strengthened as a result of the very trauma that diminished the objective beauty of her skin. Which was more important to me: My mother's patience, compassion, and wisdom or the smooth luster of unblemished skin? Beauty that appeals only to the eyes doesn't move me the way my mother's beauty moves me.

# About the Editors

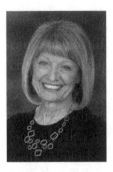

LaNae Valentine has a doctorate degree in marriage and family therapy and specializes in working with women struggling with depression, anxiety, perfectionism, body image, and eating problems. As the director of Women's Services and Resources at Brigham Young University, she is dedicated to creating programming and events that help women find their voice, recognize their worth, and realize their power for good. LaNae has presented at local and national conferences emphasizing the power we each have to create a culture that is more accepting and respectful of our diversity and uniqueness. She lives in Orem, Utah.

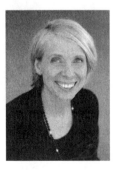

Lisa Tensmeyer Hansen is a therapist at the BYU Comprehensive Clinic and at the Provo Center for Couples and Families. She is an educational speaker on relationships, depression, anxiety, and community/family support for marginalized youth. She has been featured as the voice of mental health research on *Mormon Matters* podcasts and conducts research regarding best outcomes for young people. She and her husband, Bill, are the parents of seven children and a few extras.